The Physiology of Resistance Training

TOMMY LUNDBERG

Table of
Contents _____

THE AUTHOR'S INTRODUCTION VI

FOREWORD BY PER TESCH..VII

INTRODUCTION TO RESISTANCE TRAINING X
    A look back on history...X
    Resistance training as an exercise modality.............................. XII
    Muscle strength..XIII
    Research on the physiology of resistance training....................XIV

PART 1.   **BASIC MUSCLE PHYSIOLOGY**

CHAPTER 1.   **MUSCLE STRUCTURE AND FUNCTION**.....................................2
    The overall structure of the muscles... 3
    Muscle Arrangement.. 3
    Muscle microstructure.. 4
    Summary.. 8

CHAPTER 2.   **MUSCLE CONTRACTION AND ENERGY METABOLISM**...............10
    Fuel for exercise 11
    Neuromuscular control of movement 14
    Muscle contraction: The sliding filament theory 19
    Summary.. 20

CHAPTER 3.   **BIOLOGICAL BASIS OF FORCE PRODUCTION**............................22
    Nervous system control 23
    Muscle actions 24
    Muscle architecture... 25
    The contractile properties of the muscle fibers 26
    Mechanical relationships 27
    Force transfer 29
    Summary.. 30

CHAPTER 4.   **MUSCLE PROTEIN TURNOVER** 32
    Dynamic synthesis and degradation... 33
    Methods for measuring protein turnover.................................. 33
    Muscle protein metabolism during resistance training.............. 35
    Summary.. 38

PART 2.   ADAPTATIONS TO RESISTANCE TRAINING

CHAPTER 5.   NEUROMUSCULAR ADAPTATIONS..40
Strength gains..41
Neural adaptations..42
Agonist activation..43
Neuromuscular Inhibition..46
Rate of force development...47
Summary..48

CHAPTER 6.   HYPERTROPHY...49
Measuring muscle hypertrophy..50
Time course of hypertrophy...51
Hyperplasia..52
Hypertrophy of individual fibers...53
Difference between muscle groups...56
Effect of age..56
Selective hypertrophy in different muscle groups.....................................56
Individual variation in hypertrophy...57
Does muscle hypertrophy causally determine strength development? 59
Summary..59

CHAPTER 7.   MECHANISMS FOR HYPERTROPHY 61
Stimuli for muscle hypertrophy..62
The acute cellular response to resistance training....................................65
Molecular regulation of protein turnover 65
Satellite cell activation and myonuclei accretion......................................69
Regulation of protein breakdown 71
Summary of established and emerging mechanisms..................................71
Summary..72

CHAPTER 8.   METABOLIC AND HORMONAL ADAPTATIONS...............................74
Acute metabolic response to resistance training 75
Long-term adaptations...75
Hormonal adaptations...77
Summary..80

CHAPTER 9.   MUSCLE ARCHITECTURE, BONE, AND ELASTIC COMPONENTS 81

Muscle architecture 82

The elastic components 85

Bone tissue 86

Summary 87

PART 3.   DETERMINANTS OF RESISTANCE TRAINING OUTCOMES

CHAPTER 10.   TRAINING VARIABLES AND PROGRAM DESIGN 90

General training principles 91

Training variables 91

Periodization 98

Time of day 99

Different types of exercise 100

Summary 102

CHAPTER 11.   THE ROLE OF PROTEIN INTAKE 104

Protein needs 105

Optimization of protein synthesis during resistance training 105

The importance of protein timing 107

Protein consumption prior to sleep 108

Summary 109

CHAPTER 12.   DIETARY SUPPLEMENTS FOR RESISTANCE TRAINING 110

Definition of dietary supplements 111

Why use supplements? 111

Which dietary supplements work? 112

Risks and disadvantages of dietary supplements 113

Summary 114

CHAPTER 13.   MUSCLE FATIGUE AND EXERCISE-INDUCED MUSCLE DAMAGE 115

Muscle fatigue 116

Exercise-induced muscle damage 118

Summary 120

Contents

CHAPTER 14. RECOVERY STRATEGIES **122**

    Cold-water immersion..123

    Antioxidants...123

    Anti-inflammatory drugs...124

    Compression garments...125

    Summary...125

CHAPTER 15. CONCURRENT RESISTANCE AND ENDURANCE TRAINING **127**

    Background to research on concurrent training 128

    Effects of concurrent training on muscle hypertrophy 129

    Effects of concurrent training on maximal strength and power 130

    Resistance training for endurance performance 132

    Summary...134

CHAPTER 16. HEALTH BENEFITS OF RESISTANCE TRAINING **135**

    Resistance training for health 136

    Resistance training and cardiovascular health 137

    Resistance training and type-2 diabetes 137

    Resistance training for specific patient groups 138

    Resistance training and cognitive function 138

    Resistance training and bone health 138

    Resistance training for weight loss 139

    Summary...140

CHAPTER 17. RESISTANCE TRAINING FOR SPECIFIC TARGET GROUPS..........................**141**

    Resistance training for the elderly 142

    Resistance training for children and adolescents................................145

    Sex aspects in resistance training...146

    Resistance training during pregnancy 148

    Resistance training for athletes 149

    Summary...151

FIGURE REFERENCES...**152**

REFERENCES **154**

The Author's Introduction

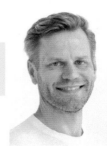

While there is an abundance of books on resistance training that cover everything from anatomy to detailed exercise programs, this book offers a fresh perspective. It seeks to explore the underlying physiology that explains the typical results and adaptations associated with resistance training, particularly muscle hypertrophy and strength gains.

The book is structured like a textbook and is intended for students and professionals in the fields of sports, medicine, and health sciences. However, I hope that it is equally valuable to sports and health professionals, coaches, and anyone interested in the fundamental physiology of resistance training. A basic understanding of exercise physiology, whether through formal education or independent research, is beneficial for the reader to fully appreciate the content.

This is not a typical guidebook packed with training programs. On the contrary, it aims to provide a comprehensive understanding of the physiological underpinnings of resistance training. The scientific approach of this book is intended to enhance the reader's ability to absorb and critically analyze the vast information available today in the field of muscle physiology and resistance training. The text draws practical parallels to training principles and program design only where it makes a clear connection to the physiology discussed.

After an introductory first chapter, the book unfolds in three sections. The first section highlights basic muscle physiology, which is central to understanding muscle force production and training adaptations in the form of muscle hypertrophy and enhanced strength. The second section addresses specific adaptations to resistance training, focusing on muscle hypertrophy.

The book culminates in the third part, where I examine various factors that influence or are closely related to the effects of resistance training. Topics such as muscle fatigue, recovery, muscle soreness, the role of protein and supplements, and the effects of various training variables on training response are explored. In addition, the health benefits and biological sex aspects of resistance training are discussed, as well as special considerations for specific groups such as adolescents, seniors, pregnant women, and athletes.

Throughout the book, relevant scientific articles are cited when they add to the discussion, especially when discussing the results of specific studies. Since it is impossible to mention all the respected researchers in the field of resistance training, I do not claim that this book is comprehensive in this regard. I welcome feedback on the content of the book. Feel free to reach out on social media! I hope to see future editions of the book.

I am grateful to everyone who has given me feedback on specific sections of the book, as well as to the fellow researchers who collaborated on the original Swedish version of this book. A special thanks to Per Tesch, my PhD mentor, for introducing me to the academic world and for generously sharing some history lessons and great anecdotes in the foreword.

TOMMY LUNDBERG
Stockholm, September 2023

Foreword by Per Tesch

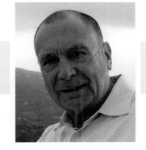

When Tommy approached me to write this foreword, my mind immediately turned to the evolving definition of resistance training. I could have delved into the details, but instead I felt compelled to describe the transformative journey of resistance training, which I have been intimately intertwined with. My passion for sport led to a lifelong pursuit that culminated in conducting numerous resistance training studies, many of which I am proud to have managed alongside dedicated colleagues and students.

In my early years involved with sports, barbells and dumbbells was for Olympic weightlifters, power lifters, bodybuilders, football players, serious track athletes and perhaps a few more. As a competitive flat-water kayaker, we did scattered training with light weights off season. During my two college years as a physical education student, we had two hours dedicated to strength training classes. Somewhat at my surprise and unprepared, I was asked by our teacher to run the classes together with a fellow kayaker. The "exercise physiology" research field was shaped by giants like Per–Olof Åstrand and Bengt Saltin, with roots in endurance training. Exercise physiology was essentially all about aerobic exercise. Who could image back then, that soccer players, cross–country skiers, not to mention golfers, would engage in systematic resistance training?

I completed my doctoral thesis on fatigue and lactic acid accumulation in fast and slow twitch muscle fibers during short–term, intense exercise (Acta Physiol Scand. 1980). My supervisor at the Karolinska Institute was the dynamic and creative Jan Karlsson. While focusing on questions relevant to anaerobic work, training and performance, a review paper by Keul and co–workers (Medicine & Science in Sports and Exercise 1978) had caught my eyes and subsequently intrigued me to investigate muscle metabolism during acute resistance exercise (Eur J Appl Physiol. 55:362–366, 1986). The authors had bluntly claimed that the stores of ATP and creatine phosphate would sufficiently fuel muscle during resistance–type exercise. This may be true for a competitive weightlifter, but hardly for a bodybuilder carrying out 4 sets of 10 repetitions and several consecutive exercises targeting the same muscle group. Hence, we recruited some of the best bodybuilders and conducted the experiments at a local Gym in Stockholm. Analyses of repeated biopsy samples showed that all energy systems, including lipolysis and glycogenolysis, were heavily used. Our finding that stores of muscle triglycerides, and similar to heavy aerobic exercise, are depleted during 30 minutes of resistance training (four sets each of front and back squats, knee extensions, and the leg press) raised a few eyebrows (Eur J Appl Physiol. 61: 5–10, 1990).

My post–doc year at the US Army Research Institute of Environmental Medicine, Natick near Boston, allowed me to test my own wings. Several of my research fellows and friends at the Natick lab had backgrounds as bodybuilders, powerlifters or weightlifters. Together we explored how "muscle profile" features (e.g., fiber type composition, fiber size, capillarization, enzyme activity etc.) correlated with all types of physical performance (e.g., maximal strength, explosiveness, muscle endurance) in field soldiers.

At the time there was an increased awareness of skeletal muscle plasticity and the early onset of neuromuscular adaptations that occurs in response to activity or inactivity. Unfortunately, our study of extreme endurance athletes who were forced to refrain from training for extended periods of time due to injury or illness and became significantly stronger, was never published. To weightlifters and sprinters, it was already known that endurance training is "bad news" as it could readily compromise strength, speed and explosiveness. The knowledge and experience I had gained now was the foundation and gateway to an "Exercise Physiology" research career with focus on resistance training.

When the chief medical officer of the Royal Swedish Air Force called, I decided to return to Stockholm and the Karolinska Institute. Research funds had been allocated to investigate whether resistance training (calf, thigh and abdominal muscles) could serve as an aid to improve G-tolerance in fighter pilots during aerial combat. The hypothesis was that by strengthening lower body muscles, blood pooling in the legs would be reduced, preventing a serious drop in blood pressure potentially resulting in "grey out" or unconsciousness. Our experiments in the human centrifuge showed that a rather modest resistance training program in fact improved G-tolerance (Aviat Space Envir Med 54: 691–695, 1983). I believe this most significant effect was due to neural adaptations rather than muscle hypertrophy. The publication received global attention and very soon fighter pilots around the world had their own gyms.

The ignorance of resistance training as a mean to improve fitness was monumental among leading sports physicians and researchers at the time. "Strength training causes hypertension," trumpeted one professor and devoted long-distance runner. Thus, we decided to compare blood pressure in medical students and 31 bodybuilders (Can J Appl Sport Sci 13: 31–34, 1988). As is turned out, the bodybuilders possessed normal resting blood pressure and significantly less cardiac stress during light to heavy exercise, and greater work and oxygen uptake capacity than the healthy and rather fit medical students.

In an almost virgin research field, it was inspiring, encouraging and rewarding to engage in studies of acute and chronic responses to weight training, and all its potential applications for improving athletic performance – not to mention preventing and treating disease. For many serious diagnoses, the "doctor's order" back then, was caution or a ban on exercise. Today resistance training is prescribed as medicine!

For years there was a misguided discussion about eccentric exercise as it was believed to cause damaging muscle soreness and hence should be implemented with caution. "No Pain – No Gain" and "Negative Reps" "Forced Reps" etc., had been preached in muscle magazines since the 1950's. Could it be that generations of "plate heads" had been wrong? Of course not, but perhaps it was the moment to reassess the importance of eccentric actions in resistance training?

At the time of my dissertation, I was introduced to Professor Paavo Komi, University of Jyväskylä, Finland. He became a mentor, friend, research partner, and a great source of inspiration to me. Komi and associates conducted groundbreaking applied studies on the importance of the "stretch-shortening cycle," i.e., how concentric and eccentric actions work in synergy. As a post-doc at Penn State University, he had also published a classic paper showing that eccentric resistance training produced a more profound training response than resistance training with concentric actions only (Ergonomics 15: 417–434, 1972). The work was almost forgotten, and we engineered a motorized ergometer and performed a series of experiments in an effort to distinguish neural and muscular effects after isokinetic concentric and eccentric exercise. Komi's results were confirmed (Acta Physiol Scand 140: 31–39, 1990). However, muscle hypertrophy after eccentric isokinetic training was modest. This finding changed my view on the effectiveness of isokinetic training.

Dr. Paul Buchanan was a young physician and Med Ops at NASA who cared for the very first "the Original Seven" astronauts in the 1960's (see Tom Clancy's "The Right Stuff"). When Buchanan recruited me to NASA's Kennedy Space Center in Florida in the late 1980's, he was ultimately medically responsible for the health of the astronauts. My popular science articles in Joe Weider's Muscle & Fitness, which Paul subscribed to, and the published results of my studies on fighter pilots brought me, extremely flattered and proud, and Paul together. At age of +60, Paul Buchanan was dedicated to resistance training. At that time, given his age and professional status at NASA, he was considered somewhat aloof for prioritizing his daily strength training routine and a protein shake over a business lunch. Buchanan struggled to convince his colleagues and administrators at NASA that resistance training, but not endurance training, builds muscle. It was already believed muscle atrophy occurred during prolonged space travel. Yet, it was hard for him to make the sell that resistance training must be the sole in-flight method to counteract muscle atrophy.

This was in the aftermath of the tragic Challenger accident (seven astronauts had died in an explosion shortly after launch). For several years the Space Shuttle program was on hold. Paul and I shared the idea of finding a solution to "lift weights" in the absence of gravity. Along with blessed and talented friend and colleague Dr. Gary Dudley, we sat out on the mission. Initially, we designed and employed various unloading models (simulating the conditions in space) to assess various aspects of skeletal muscle atrophy of the postural calf and thigh muscles (J Appl Physiol:70:1882–1885, 1991). In parallel we ran studies addressing the importance of concentric and eccentric muscle actions in resistance training (Acta Physiol Scand 143: 177–185, 1991). The results were intended to shed light on how we could develop technology to replace dumbbells and barbells for resistance training in a zero–gravity environment. It soon became evident eccentric muscle actions must be used for effective, time–efficient, low energy cost, in–flight training.

I experienced some wonderful years at Cape Canaveral and Cocoa Beach in the environment that was breathing space. On any day, I could feel the wings of history from 60's Apollo. At Kennedy Space Center, Hans Berg and I conducted the very first experiments using the YoYo Leg Press (A Gravity–Independent Ergometer to be Used for Resistance Training in Space; Aviat Space Environ Med 65: 752–756, 1994). By means of functional magnetic resonance imaging (fMRI), we showed muscle involvement was much greater compared with barbell squats. Additional experimental data generated by means of fMRI were published in the book Muscle Meets Magnet (published later by Human Kinetics and entitled Target Bodybuilding), which details muscle involvement for numerous established arm and leg exercises.

It is mind blowing how much has been achieved from the early 1990's until now, to understand and appreciate the benefits of resistance training. Certainly, progress and development of methods and break–through technologies have produced impressive tools, for example, to study muscle from the gene level to whole muscle. While academic and more applied research have been of great significance to define resistance training, it is nevertheless the marketplace; the fitness and healthcare industries, and talented entrepreneurs who have been the driving forces responsible for the boom in people of both sexes and all ages taking part in, and entertaining resistance training.

I aimed at completing the long–term goals that our Kennedy Space Center team had shared with passion. In 1999–2001 I conducted the study that had been on my mind since the years at Kennedy Space Center. With a 3–year grant from NASA, men and women were subjected to unilateral lower limb unloading while performing YoYo quad exercises 2–3 times a week over five weeks to combat muscle atrophy. To our surprise they even packed on muscle despite being unloaded 24 hours a day (J Appl Physiol 96: 1451–1458, 2004). A few years later, in Toulouse in France, we studied men and women who were bedridden for up to 90 days and had them do resistance training on a YoYo Multi–Gym (Eur J Appl Physiol 93: 294–305, 2004). It worked! Together with the Russian Space Agency in Moscow, we locked up prospective cosmonauts in a small space capsule for 110 days to study compliance, injury risk, and exercise adaptation (Eur J Appl Physiol 90: 44–49, 2003). Finally, after many years of research and development and "red tape," NASA and ESA launched and installed the YoYo Multi–Gym on the International Space Station. At home, we have successfully applied the YoYo technique to elite athletes and various patient populations (Front Physio 18: 1–16, 2017).

Tommy's book, which you are about to entertain, serves an important function. There are countless writings and now internet forums, apps and podcasts that give tips on exercises and workout programs. Today, a search and programs and instructions are just a click away. This book summarizes and contains the collected and latest knowledge on the physiology of resistance training. It serves as a guide and offers inspiration for the resistance training program you want to use, or perhaps confirm that you are on the right track. It is as relevant to the student as it is to the athlete, teacher, coach, personal trainer, health care provider or clinician. Do not expect Tommy to give you solutions and ready–made recipes for successful resistance training – that's your job!

PER TESCH
Retired professor

Introduction to Resistance Training

A LOOK BACK ON HISTORY

The ability to generate extraordinary muscular strength has always fascinated mankind, and various forms of strength and physique competitions have been around for a very long time. Dating back to 2500 BC, illustrations of various strength competitions have been found in Egyptian tombs [1]. Much later, but still several centuries before our era, Greek soldiers performed strengthening exercises using the human body as resistance.

The application of the resistance training principles of overload and progression dates back to ancient Greece and the mythical Milo of Croton (born 550 B.C.), who is said to have carried a bull on his shoulders from birth to adulthood. One of the earliest forms of bodybuilding competition was found in the Greek city of Sparta, where men posed naked and were judged on their bodily physique.

More modern medical anatomy developed in the 16th and 17th centuries. It laid the foundation for understanding the structure and function of the musculoskeletal system. Muscular fitness was already valued at this time, as noted in one of Benjamin Franklin's writings in 1786. He noted that he had valued training with dumbbells for over 14 years [2].

Physical exercise with one's own body prevailed into the 19th century, most notably with Per Henrick Ling, the Swedish father of gymnastics, in the forefront. During the same period, Gustaf Zander invented the prototype for the gyms we visit today. He constructed equipment out of wood, with weights, levers, and springs that offered resistance. Zander gave individual instructions on how long and how much each piece of equipment should be used, just as today's personal trainer prescribes workouts. The first Zander Institute opened in Stockholm in 1865, and both men and women were welcome to train. Zander was driven by a strong desire to improve people's energy and health and to "with steam save the sick society", as he reportedly put it [3]. The Zander Institutes later became a global success and new facilities opened around the world.

In the early 1900s, there was virtually no research on resistance training, but important experiments were conducted that improved our understanding of basic muscle physiological principles. In the 1920s–1930s, AV Hill studied the contractility of skeletal muscle at various loads and speeds (the force–velocity relationship) [4], and the muscle contraction mechanism, now known as the sliding filament theory, was introduced in the 1950s by Andrew Huxley [5].

Prior to the 1950s, studies of resistance training were scarce in the medical literature. As James Nuzzo notes in his historical review, 339 studies on resistance training were documented between 1894 and 1979 [6]. Remarkably, only 17 of these studies were published before 1950.

The positive effects of resistance training began to be noted in the scientific literature after World War II. This was largely due to Thomas DeLorme, an army doctor, who had noted the long rehabilitation time for various musculoskeletal injuries suffered by American soldiers. He decided to experiment with a new rehabilitation technique that involved 10 maximum repetitions over multiple sets. DeLorme called the method "Progressive Resistance Exercise [7]," and he was the first to use the term "repetition maximum" (RM) as a reference point for loading. The new rehabilitation method was very successful and led to resistance training research finally picking up steam.

Dr. Richard A. Berger was one of the first to study the effects of various sets, loads, and repetitions on the development of strength. In his 1962 study, "Effect of Varied Weight Training Programs on Strength," sets and repetitions were systematically varied to determine if and how they affected strength development [8].

One early contributor, Philip Rash, does not receive as much recognition in the literature as contemporaries such as DeLorme and Berger. Rash appears to be the pioneer who studied both the effects of resistance training on mental health and the combined effects of resistance training and protein supplementation on muscle size and strength. Like many other researchers of his time, Rash found that the observed increase in muscle size was not the primary cause of improved muscle strength. He also studied the benefits of resistance training for the mentally ill and documented the effects of such training on patients in a neuropsychiatric setting. Interestingly, according to James Nuzzo [6], this research has not been cited.

In the 1950s, interest grew. Hettinger and Muller wrote several influential articles on resistance training methods. In a 1959 article, Muller described these observations, some of which are recognized today, while others have been debunked [9]:

- Inactivity can reduce strength by about 30% in a week, but this loss can be quickly recovered when activity is resumed.
- Muscle atrophy can be halted by a single daily contraction at one-fifth of maximum strength.
- To maintain a normal level of strength, contractions should be between one-fifth and one-third of maximum strength.
- The ability of muscles to increase maximum strength varies depending on the muscle and the individual. In men, it peaks at age 25 and halves by ages 10 and 60.
- The rate of strength gain is twice as high in men as in women.
- This ability to increase strength is minimal in winter, but peaks in summer. It is enhanced by ultraviolet radiation. A high-protein diet does not enhance it, but a low-protein diet may decrease it.

Neural adaptations to resistance training were studied beginning in the 1970s. This was preceded by fundamental findings in the 1950s on the recruitment pattern of motor units by Elwood Henneman, now known as **Henneman's size principle** [10]. The 1979 study by Moritani and deVries is the most widely cited research paper from the period up to the 1980s [11]. It examined the sequence of neural and muscular responses to resistance training. The authors theorized that the strength gains observed in the first 4 weeks of a training program were primarily due to neural adaptations. The strength gains after this period were attributed to muscle hypertrophy.

Throughout the 20th century, more and more equipment were invented, from free weights, dumbbells, and barbells to today's fitness equipment, which became increasingly popular beginning in the 1970s. In the United States, fitness promoters such as Joe Weider and Jack Lalanne, who were active in the mid-20th century, spread information and knowledge about fitness and bodybuilding. By the mid-20th century, it was primarily enthusiasts in the fitness industry, along with various publishers and weight manufacturers, who ensured that knowledge about resistance training and its effects was disseminated [2].

For a long time, the prevailing view was that resistance training could be harmful to health because of the rapid changes in blood pressure that occur during strength exercises. In recent decades, this view has been revised and today the positive health effects of resistance training are increasingly recognized.

The number of published scientific articles on resistance training increased almost exponentially from 1970 to 2010 [2]. Much of the research in the early 1980s addressed the basic function and energy metabolism of muscle fibers during acute exercise and chronic resistance training. The mechanisms of muscle fatigue began to be studied in detail, and the effects of different training programs and exercise choices were compared. Robert Staron was another pioneer who conducted several important studies in the 1990s that expanded our knowledge of muscle fiber adaptations to training in both men and women.

In the last 20 years, molecular biology research has received more attention due to rapid technological development. This research gained even more momentum after the mapping of the human genome was completed in the early 2000s. In the last few decades, gym culture and the fitness industry have grown. Resistance training is now considered a central part of the training program for both athletes and people training for general health and fitness.

RESISTANCE TRAINING AS AN EXERCISE MODALITY

Most people associate resistance training with relatively heavy weights lifted a few times *(repetitions)* over a number of series *(sets)* per muscle group. The most established competitive forms of strength and physique are weightlifting, powerlifting, and bodybuilding. Weightlifting debuted as an Olympic sport in 1896. Today, there are two different forms of competition in Olympic weightlifting: snatch and the clean and jerk. In the clean and jerk, the barbell is lifted from the floor to the extended arms over the head, while in the snatch, the barbell is rotated from the floor to the shoulders and then over the head. Both lifts involve multiple joints and illustrate the high demands on technique and strength associated with many complex resistance exercises.

Powerlifting is about lifting as much weight as possible in three different lifts: squat, bench press, and deadlift. In bodybuilding, muscle mass is the primary goal, both in terms of size, shape, and appearance. Some of the training methods long used by bodybuilders are still the basis for the advice generally given to recreational athletes seeking to maximize muscle growth.

Resistance training today includes a variety of training methods with and without the use of equipment and machines. Training with free weights (dumbbells and barbells) and machines is still a central component, but other equipment such as kettlebells, rubber bands, and balance balls are also widely used. Yet, resistance training using your own body is still viable. The term *"functional training"* has evolved into a concept to describe more complex exercises, with or without weights, that focus on developing strength, flexibility, and coordination in specific movements rather than muscle strength or muscle mass for isolated muscle groups.

The classic resistance training program using heavy weights lifted relatively infrequently is quite different from traditional endurance training, where the total volume of exercise is large, but the absolute force generated by each muscular action (for example, a running stride) is relatively small. Strength and endurance training in their pure forms are therefore located at either end of a training continuum (Fig. 0.1).

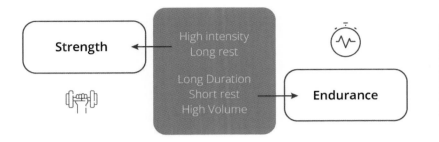

Figure 0.1.
Strength and endurance are considered at each end of the training continuum. Specific training forms are often classified based on intensity, duration, length of rest periods, and total volume.

Recently, training modalities that challenge this traditional dogma have gained popularity. Repeated sprint-interval training, often performed on a stationary bike, is similar to resistance training in terms of high intensity performed for a limited time (often 30 seconds or less). However, this form of training is still primarily associated with improved cardiovascular fitness. It has also become increasingly apparent that low-load resistance training can result in significant muscle growth and strength gains when performed close to failure, while also improving muscular endurance. This challenges the traditional textbook view that the effects of endurance and resistance training are vastly different or even antagonistic.

As our knowledge of the molecular response of the skeletal muscle to exercise has increased, it has also become increasingly clear that many of the signals triggered by exercise are the same for endurance, sprint, and resistance training. Several prominent muscle adaptations to training are therefore common to these types of training, although the magnitude of each of these adaptations can be strongly influenced by the manipulation of training variables such as intensity, duration, and rest time.

There has also been an increase in the popularity of training forms that require endurance and strength simultaneously. This highlights the complexity of training. In the future, it may be that the traditional classification of training modalities, such as aerobic and anaerobic training or resistance and endurance training, will be less static.

MUSCLE STRENGTH

Muscle strength is usually defined as the maximum force that can be produced by a muscle or group of muscles against resistance. The term **muscle function** is often used to refer to either the maximum muscle strength during a particular task or the muscle force in relation to the size of the muscle (**specific force**). Specific force is often expressed as the force divided by the cross-sectional area of the muscle. Specific force can vary between different muscles and different people, but can be estimated at around 20 N/cm [12].

Muscle strength is often measured in absolute terms by **isometric testing, isokinetic testing,** or by using free weights or machines to determine the maximum load that can be lifted once (1RM). Isokinetic force measurements measure muscle force at various joint angular velocities ranging from zero (isometric) to velocities greater than 300 angular degrees per second, which is about one-third of what humans can produce during maximal knee extension.

Isokinetic means that the velocity is constant during the force measurement. An advantage of these tests is that force production is measured throughout the range of motion, making it possible to pinpoint specific phases of the movement. These tests are also safe and easy to perform, even for individuals with little experience in resistance training. Isokinetic testing is often used in the context of rehabilitation, where the goal is to track muscle strength recovery after an injury. The reproducibility of the measurements is relatively high, which makes these tests very useful in research studies as well.

A test of maximal isometric force in an isokinetic dynamometer is called **maximal voluntary isometric contraction** (MVIC), which is considered the reference method for measuring muscle strength in research studies. The downside is that the MVIC test requires specialized equipment that most people do not have access to. It is also important to consider that many "real-world" movements or sport-specific actions consist of dynamic and more complex movements that cannot be tested with this type of equipment.

With free weights or weight stack machines, it is common to measure **maximum strength**, i.e., 1RM (1 repetition maximum), the weight that can only be lifted once. The disadvantage of the 1RM test is that many free weight exercises require good technique, which means that this form of testing is only suitable for people who have previous experience with the specific exercises tested. In many research studies, various hand dynamometers are used to estimate grip strength. This general measure of muscle strength has been shown to correlate with many different biological functions and with health status, life expectancy, and the risk of suffering from serious diseases.

To estimate **explosive strength** (the ability to generate high muscle force quickly), force plates or simpler vertical jumps are used. Jump height can be used directly as an outcome measure or converted to an estimate of power development. More advanced measures of explosive strength, such as in research contexts, involve measuring the **rate of force development**. In measuring the rate of force development, the increase in force development is recorded over time during a maximal contraction. The faster the force curve rises, the higher the rate of force development.

A term often used synonymously with explosive strength in the context of resistance training is **power**. Power is defined as work per unit time or force × velocity. At maximal effort, power is clearly related to explosive strength, but by definition, power can also refer to the ability to maintain a high level of force output for an extended period of time, which is more related to **muscular endurance** (the ability to sustain a submaximal load for as long as possible).

The term **reactive force** is used to denote the ability to produce force rapidly in the transition from a decelerating **eccentric** muscle action to the subsequent **concentric** action. This ability is dependent on what is known as the **stretch-shortening cycle,** which involves active stretching of the muscle in the eccentric phase, and using elastic energy stored in the tendon and connective tissue to increase force during the subsequent concentric phase. This skill, which can be trained in various types of jumps and change-of-direction exercises, is an important part of many athletes' training programs.

RESEARCH ON THE PHYSIOLOGY OF RESISTANCE TRAINING

Methods for assessing muscle function and adaptations to resistance training are constantly being refined. The most basic knowledge about muscle work, fiber types, and nervous system regulation was gained many decades ago. In fact, in some of these areas, we know only marginally more today than we did when the breakthrough findings were made. When Andrew Huxley presented his model of how muscle contracts in the 1950s, he emphasized that the theory still did not fully explain the eccentric muscle action. Even today, 70 years later, there are gaps in our understanding of the eccentric muscle action.

The area in which the greatest progress has been made is clearly in the field of molecular biology, where researchers now have access to knowledge and methods of analysis that were almost unimaginable a few decades ago. There were high hopes among researchers that these new techniques would very quickly lead to major advances in knowledge that would make it possible to create training prescriptions specifically tailored to each individual. However, this has proved difficult, and there are still no definitive answers to fundamental questions such as why the training response varies greatly between individuals or what mechanisms cause some to lose significantly more muscle mass than others in disease or aging.

Research methods

Contemporary research on the physiology of resistance training often uses a combination of different methods and study designs to advance knowledge in specific areas. In **observational studies** (which include **epidemiological studies**), no active action is taken by the research participant. Instead, participants are observed under prevailing circumstances and the occurrence of an outcome variable is examined in relation to the data collected, for example, through surveys. The relationships between these factors are then examined. Another form of observational study is **cross-sectional studies** that compare different populations on a single occasion. An example might be a study comparing muscle mass between old and young people.

In **intervention studies**, participants are exposed to some form of intervention or treatment. A common form of intervention studies related to resistance training are randomized controlled training trials, such as comparing the effects of two different training programs or evaluating the effects of a nutritional supplement. When possible, a placebo control is included. In short-term (acute) trials, two or more interventions are studied in a so-called cross-over design. This means that each study participant performs all the interventions/tests, but in a different order. In this type of study, each subject is his or her own control, which increases the possibility of statistically detecting small differences between the different test conditions.

Basic measures of muscle size and strength remain key outcome measures, for example, to provide answers about which strength exercises are most effective. Depending on the mechanism being studied, these outcome measures are often combined with molecular analysis of muscle biopsies, more controlled experiments in animal models, or using muscle cells isolated from muscle biopsies or developed in cell culture.

Models in humans

Resistance training is the only effective loading model that can be used to study muscle hypertrophy in humans. However, one problem in the research context is that there is a wide variation in how different individuals respond to the same resistance training program. Nevertheless, human studies are necessary to test hypotheses about muscle hypertrophy that have emerged from other models of muscle growth, such as cell culture or animal studies. Alternatively, the researcher may have made interesting findings in human muscle biopsies and would like to investigate these mechanisms further in controlled cell experiments. If the focus is on more functional adaptations to resistance training, studies in humans are necessary.

Animal models

Much of the mechanistic information about muscle growth (hypertrophy) and breakdown (atrophy) comes from animal models such as mouse or rat studies. The great advantage of animal models is that many factors can be controlled. The genetic pool of laboratory mice is much less variable than in humans. Food intake and physical activity can also be much better controlled in animal models. Another advantage is that it is possible to study a whole muscle, whereas in humans, one is often forced to rely on information from a muscle biopsy taken at one or a few time points.

To induce muscle growth in animal models, various methods are used, such as stretching models, elimination of synergistic muscles, or various forms of overload protocols (mimicking resistance training in humans). All these models have their advantages and disadvantages, and the choice of method ultimately depends on the research question. However, it is inevitable that experiments in animal models can never fully resemble experiments in humans.

Isolated fibers and cell cultures

The contractile properties of muscle can be studied in detail in single muscle cells isolated from muscle biopsies or grown in a laboratory setting (myotubes). In such models, it is easy to control the environment of the muscle cells and manipulate individual variables in a controlled manner. By placing an isolated fiber (prepared from muscle tissue) in a device that measures force, the rate of shortening and force production can be studied in detail. It is also common to dissolve the muscle membrane of individual muscle cells to gain access to the environment inside the cell.

There are several drawbacks to studies of isolated fibers, the most notable being the absence of the nervous system and all extracellular components (e.g., tendons and bone). When the goal is to study intact fibers running the entire length of the fascicle, mouse or rat models are typically used. However, in humans, intact fibers have been isolated from the intercostal muscles (between the ribs) in the context of lung surgery [13]. Significant differences in calcium handling have been demonstrated in intact fibers compared to those produced in the laboratory setting (myotubes). This is an important consideration when interpreting findings obtained exclusively from cultured muscle cells.

Much of our basic knowledge of how muscle fibers are formed, developed, and remodeled comes from cell cultures. In cell cultures, muscle cells are grown from their earliest stage (stem cells) to complete myotubes. However, cultured muscle cells lack several key properties found in intact muscle fibers, and the physiological arrangement of the contractile units is not fully developed. Blood vessels are also absent, which means that circulating factors cannot be studied in a way that mimics normal physiology.

The advantage of cell culture is again that many factors can be controlled in the experiment. It is possible to genetically manipulate the cell culture, and the environment in which the cells are grown can be tightly regulated and monitored. This is important for carefully controlled mechanistic studies. Problematically, mechanisms that result from experiments in cell cultures cannot always be replicated in an intact muscle. It is also very difficult to mimic a stimulus like resistance training in cell culture.

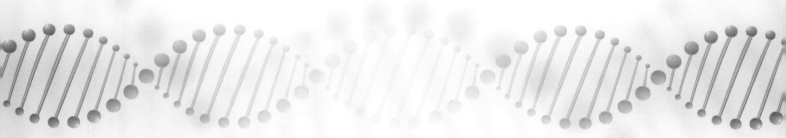

PART 1

BASIC MUSCLE PHYSIOLOGY

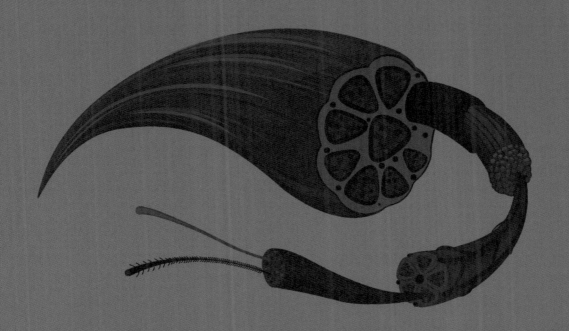

01

CHAPTER 01

MUSCLE STRUCTURE AND FUNCTION

The human musculoskeletal system consists of the skeleton, which provides stability and serves as an attachment point for muscles; the joints, which connect various bones together and thereby allow movement; and the muscles, whose contractions produce the muscular force that causes movement. In addition, the musculoskeletal system indirectly includes the nervous system that controls our voluntary movements. At the tissue level, the musculoskeletal system consists of various supporting tissues (bone tissue, connective tissue, and cartilage) and the mechanically active skeletal muscle tissue.

The human body has over 600 skeletal muscles that can account for 40–60% of total body weight in healthy adults. Skeletal muscles generate the force needed for body movements and to maintain an upright posture. In addition, muscle contractions generate heat, which helps to regulate temperature. Muscles also have a critical role in metabolism and interact with several organ systems in regulating various body functions. This chapter focuses on the general structure and function of skeletal muscle. This knowledge is fundamental to understanding how muscles function during exercise and how muscular adaptations occur in response to mechanical loading.

THE OVERALL STRUCTURE OF THE MUSCLES

Skeletal muscles are made up of many individual muscle cells called muscle fibers. Muscle fibers are formed by the fusion of several immature muscle cells. Muscle fibers differ from most other cell types in that they are shaped like a cylinder and can be very long (Fig. 1.1).

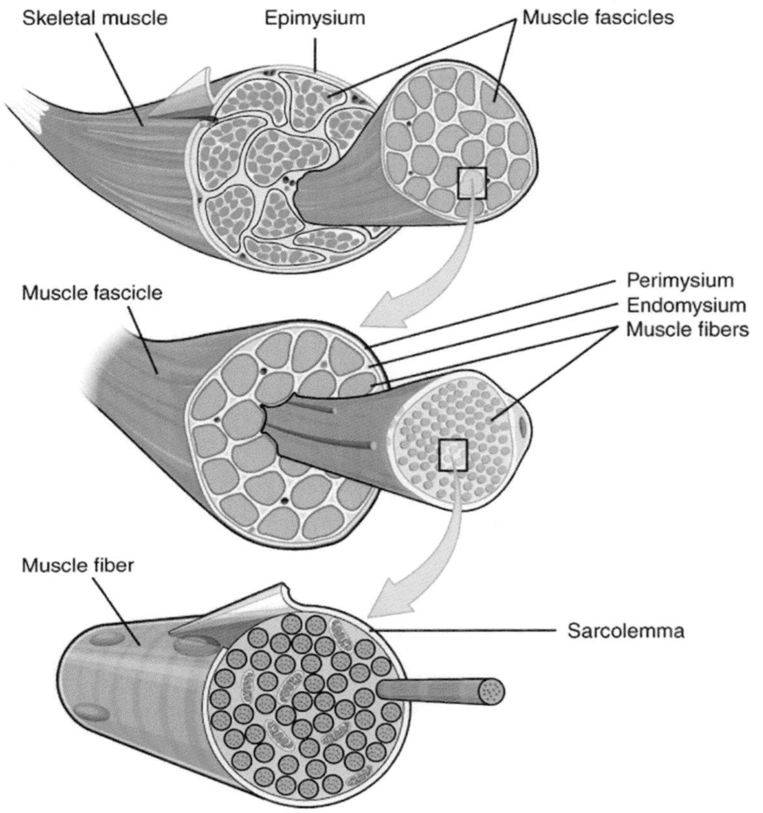

Figure 1.1.
The overall structure of the muscle. Revised from OpenStax. The complete reference can be found in the Figure references section at the end of the book.

A connective tissue layer called **endomysium** surrounds each muscle fiber along with a thin layer called **basal lamina**. An additional layer of connective tissue (**perimysium**) surrounds a group of muscle fibers, thereby dividing the muscle into distinct muscle bundles (**fascicles**). Surrounding the entire muscle is additional connective tissue called the **epimysium** or **fascia**. Various other types of cells and tissues are also found in and around the muscle, such as blood vessels, immune cells, and sensory and motor nerves.

The muscles and connective tissue are connected to the skeletal bones by tendons. The proximal tendon (closest to the center of the body) is called the origin, and the distal tendon (away from the center of the body) is called the insertion. As the muscle contracts, it shortens, and the origin and insertion approach each other. This shortening contraction is called a concentric muscle action. However, the muscle can also lengthen during the contraction, which is called the eccentric muscle action.

MUSCLE ARRANGEMENT

Skeletal muscles are usually arranged to surround a joint. Muscles that decrease the joint angle are called **flexors**, while muscles that increase the joint angle are called **extensors**. Flexors and extensors work together over a joint to decrease or increase the joint angle. An example of this principle is a regular knee extension. The quadriceps muscle group is activated to increase the knee angle, while the hamstring muscles on the back of the thigh are passively stretched, allowing the joint angle to increase. The active muscle group responsible for the primary movement is called the **agonist** (in this example, the quadriceps), while the passive muscle group is called the **antagonist** (in this case, the hamstrings). Other muscles that contribute to the movement and provide stability to the joint are called **synergists and stabilizers.**

The arrangement of muscle fibers varies greatly between different muscles (Fig. 1.2). Some muscles have a fusiform/parallel organization in which the individual fibers are more or less parallel to the anatomical direction, i.e., in line with the origin and insertion. An example of such a muscle is the elbow flexor biceps brachii. The advantage of this type of arrangement of the fibers is that the force generated acts directly on the origin and insertion, and the speed of contraction is therefore high (pronounced change in length for a given contraction force).

However, in most muscles, the fibers are angled relative to the anatomical direction. This angle is called the pennation angle. Bipennate muscles have centrally located tendon sheaths to which the fascicles attach. The rectus femoris, which is both a hip flexor and a knee extensor, is an example of such a muscle. There are also more complicated fascicle organizations such as triangular/convergent (pectoralis major), cylindrical (tibialis anterior), and multipennate (deltoid) muscles. The importance of the pennation angle in the force production of skeletal muscles is discussed later in this book.

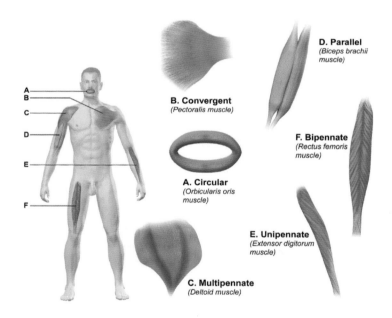

D. Parallel
(Biceps brachii muscle)

B. Convergent
(Pectoralis muscle)

F. Bipennate
(Rectus femoris muscle)

A. Circular
(Orbicularis oris muscle)

E. Unipennate
(Extensor digitorum muscle)

C. Multipennate
(Deltoid muscle)

Figure 1.2.
Different skeletal muscle types in the human body. Revised from BruceBlaus. The complete reference can be found in the Figure references section at the end of the book.

MUSCLE MICROSTRUCTURE

Notwithstanding the differences in the arrangement of the fascicles, all skeletal muscle fibers have the same microstructure. They are generally cylindrical and thin, elongated, and may sometimes run the entire length of the muscle. The muscle fibers are densely packed with very little extracellular space. The cell membrane is called the sarcolemma and the interior of the cell is called the sarcoplasm or cytoplasm. This is where all the contractile proteins and other cell organelles are located.

The contractile proteins are organized into hundreds of filamentous myofibrils that are 1–3 μm thick (Fig. 1.3). Each fiber has hundreds to thousands of individual myofibrils. The sarcoplasm also houses the nuclei, myoglobin, mitochondria, and the calcium–containing sarcoplasmic reticulum. Muscle contraction is initiated when calcium is released from the sarcoplasmic reticulum. The sarcoplasm also contains various metabolic enzymes involved in the regulation of energy metabolism.

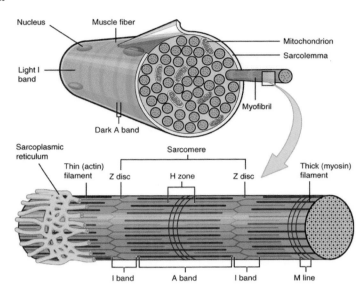

Figure 1.3.
The microstructure of the muscle fibers. Created by OpenStax. The complete reference can be found in the Figure references section at the end of the book.

A unique property of muscle fibers is that they have many nuclei per cell. Each nucleus contains the entire gene pool and expresses the genes needed to maintain the structure and function of the muscle fiber. The volume served by each nucleus is called the **myonuclear domain**. A specialized type of stem cell, called **satellite cells**, resides just below the basal lamina and remains dormant until activated by a stimulus (such as resistance training). The satellite cells can then be activated and contribute to the growth, remodeling, and repair of the cell.

Under the microscope, you can see that the muscle fibers have a striated appearance. This striation is due to the unique arrangement of the myofibrillar proteins. Along the myofibrils, dark A bands are interspersed with light I bands. In the middle of each A band is a lighter area called the H zone. This zone is only visible in a relaxed muscle. The H zone is divided by a darker line called the M line. The I bands are interrupted by zig–zag–shaped Z–discs. The Z–discs are anchor points for the contractile proteins of the myofibrils. The area between two different Z–discs defines the sarcomere. Thus, each myofibril is a long chain of sarcomeres stacked both in series and parallel to each other.

Sarcomeres are the smallest contractile units and are composed mainly of the proteins actin and myosin, which occur in thick and thin filaments. Myosin is the major protein in the thick filaments and consists of a myosin tail and myosin heads that bind to actin during contraction. The thin filament consists of actin, tropomyosin, and troponin. One end of each thin filament is anchored to a Z–disc, connecting the sarcomeres in series. Contractile proteins (mainly myosin and actin) are the most abundant proteins in muscle and account for about 85% of the fiber area in a cross–section. Other sarcoplasmic and mitochondrial proteins account for about 10% and 5% of the fiber volume, respectively [14].

The structure of sarcomeres is maintained by cytoskeletal proteins that hold the contractile proteins in place. This is done by various attachments between the myofibrils. Examples of such cytoskeletal proteins are desmin, α–actinin, vinculin, talin, and dystrophin. Another major actin–related protein is nebulin, which is thought to contribute to the length regulation of thin filaments. Between the Z–discs and the M–line, the large protein titin acts to hold myosin in place. These cytoskeletal proteins are important for force transmission in muscle, as discussed in Chapter 3.

Muscle fiber types

Skeletal muscles have different types of fibers with different contractile properties. The original basis for classifying fiber types as red and white came from visual inspection of muscle tissue in animals. Since the 1960s, when Swedes Jonas Bergström and Eric Hultman reintroduced the procedure of obtaining muscle biopsies, it has been possible to perform biochemical analyses of human muscle samples for research purposes. Such studies have clearly shown differences in muscle fiber composition and biochemical properties that can be distinguished by different laboratory methods.

By incubating a small cross-section of the muscle sample at different pH values, fiber type composition can be determined enzymatically by the activity of the enzyme myofibrillar ATPase, an enzyme that converts the energy of the ATP molecule into mechanical muscle work (contractions). High ATPase activity results in a faster contraction rate. Muscle fiber types can also be determined by using specific antibodies to stain the slow and fast isoforms of the myosin protein.

The most important functional difference between fiber types is the rate at which fibers contract and relax (Table 1.1). Three major types of motor units with associated fiber types have been identified as occurring in human muscle tissue. These fiber types are referred to as type 1, type 2A, and type 2X. Most skeletal muscles contain these three fiber types, but to varying degrees. The fiber composition thus varies between different muscles and between different people, and the distribution is largely controlled by genetic factors. It should be noted that the percentage of pure fiber type 2X is actually very low, especially in healthy people who do resistance training.

The outer thigh muscle, vastus lateralis, has a fiber type distribution corresponding to 50/50% type 1 and type 2 fibers, although large individual variations occur [15]. The inner calf muscle, soleus, consists of an even higher proportion of slow muscle fibers, while some of the upper extremity muscles may contain a higher proportion of type 2 fibers. There are also so-called hybrid fibers, which have mixed properties. These can be seen as an intermediate stage between the pure fiber types.

Human muscle fibers express the 2X isoform of the myosin protein rather than the 2B isoform, which is sometimes referred to in older textbooks and scientific articles and is found in small mammals. Fiber type has a strong influence on contraction rate and fatigue resistance, as well as the ability to grow in response to mechanical stimuli. Type 2 fibers tend to increase in size more than the slower type 1 fibers in response to resistance training.

Table 1.1.
An overview of the properties of the different fiber types.

	TYPE 1	TYPE 2A	TYPE 2X
Shortening velocity	Slow	Fast	Very fast
Force development	Low	Higher	Highest
Myofibrillar ATP degradation	Low	Higher	Highest
Activation threshold	Low	Higher	Highest

Motor unit size	Small	Larger	Largest
Mitochondrial content	High	Less	Least
Glycolytic enzyme content	Low	High	Highest
Fatigue-resistance	Very fatigue-resistant	Intermediate	Very fatigue-sensitive

Contractile properties

The slow type 1 fibers have a low maximum shortening velocity, and the relaxation time is also long. The fast fiber types, on the other hand, contract rapidly, and the relaxation time is short (Fig. 1.4). This means that the maximum power is considerably higher in the fast fibers compared to the slow fibers. When the maximum isometric force is expressed relative to the fiber area, there is a much smaller difference between fiber types. Thus, the speed of shortening is the most important discriminating factor between the different fiber types.

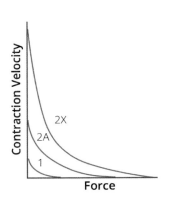
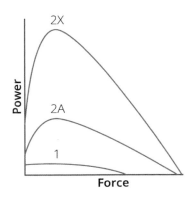

Figure 1.4.
Schematic diagram of the contractile properties of muscle fibers. The left panel shows the contraction velocity at different levels of force development. The right panel shows the power development.

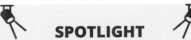

SPOTLIGHT
Why do some muscle groups respond better to resistance training than others?

· ·

Most regular gym goers have noticed that not all muscle groups respond equally well in terms of muscle growth and strength gains. An example of a muscle group that is considered difficult to train is the calf muscle. The reason for this is that the calf muscle is an important postural muscle (active when we stand upright) and is therefore built with a large proportion of slow type 1 fibers. The type 1 fibers have a growth potential that is about half that of the type 2 fibers. Therefore, a greater muscular load and effort is required to stimulate muscle hypertrophy in calf muscles. A non-postural muscle group such as the triceps muscle group on the back of the arm consists of a relatively large proportion of type 2 fibers. The anabolic response to resistance training in such a muscle group is considerably stronger.

The more pronounced red color of the slow fibers is mainly due to the high content of myoglobin. The slow fibers also have more mitochondria and capillaries than the fast fibers. The type 1 fibers also have a higher capacity for energy metabolism using oxygen (aerobic ATP production) and are much more resistant to fatigue. Type 2X fibers are generally, but not always, larger than type 1 fibers and, in addition to the difference in myosin protein composition and faster shortening speed, have a greater capacity for anaerobic breakdown of carbohydrates (glycolytic capacity) than slow fibers. Type 2A fibers are generally considered intermediate fibers, meaning they are faster than type 1 fibers, but still relatively fatigue resistant.

Although muscle fiber type is largely genetically determined, fibers are highly plastic and adapt metabolically and functionally to various stimuli, such as specific training regimens. Endurance athletes have a high percentage of type 1 fibers, while sprinters have a high percentage of type 2 fibers. The reason for this difference is likely due to genetic selection against a sport that fits a person's genetic profile, rather than long–term training alone causing the changes. Training adaptations of muscle fibers are discussed further in Chapter 6.

The plasticity of muscle fibers

Muscle fibers adapt to changes in the environment and mechanical stress and can quickly change which new proteins to produce. The information in the DNA of the nuclei is used to build these new proteins. In the first step, the information in the DNA is transferred into messenger RNA (mRNA) in a process called transcription (Fig. 1.5). The mRNA molecule is a single–stranded copy of the gene and carries the code for how the new protein should be made (i.e., the order in which the different amino acids should be combined). During the translation process, the information in the genetic code is translated into a new functional protein. The translation process takes place in the ribosomes of cells. Later in the book, it will be made clear how resistance training can affect both transcription and translation, and thus alter the protein content of fibers.

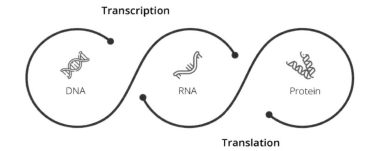

Transcription

DNA   RNA   Protein

Translation

Figure 1.5.
Transcription and translation.

SUMMARY

- ➭ Skeletal muscles produce the force needed for body movements and the maintenance of an upright posture.

- ➭ The muscles and connective tissue are connected to the skeletal bone by tendons (origin and attachment).

- ➭ Skeletal muscles are made up of many individual muscle cells called muscle fibers.

- ➭ The muscles are surrounded by a layer of connective tissue (epimysium). There is also a layer of connective tissue around each bundle of muscle fibers (perimysium) and around the individual muscle fibers (endomysium).

- ➭ A muscle contraction that results in a shortening of the muscle is called a concentric muscle action.

- ➭ Muscle contraction resulting in simultaneous lengthening of the muscle is called eccentric muscle action.

➲   Skeletal bones act as levers for skeletal muscles to pass over a joint to produce movement.

➲   The currently active muscle group that changes the joint angle is called the agonist.

➲   The passive muscle group on the other side of the joint is called the antagonist.

➲   Muscles have a different shape and architecture depending on where they are located.

➲   The interior of the muscle cell contains the sarcoplasm, nuclei, myoglobin, mitochondria, and the sarcoplasmic reticulum.

➲   The myofibrils are divided by Z–discs into the smallest functional units – the sarcomeres.

➲   Sarcomeres are the smallest contractile units and are mainly composed of the contractile proteins actin and myosin.

➲   Myosin is the thick filament that binds to actin during muscle contraction with the help of the myosin head.

➲   The thin filament actin also consists of tropomyosin and troponin, which are important proteins in muscle contraction. One end of each actin filament is attached to a Z–disc.

➲   Skeletal muscles have different types of fibers with different contractile properties, type 1, type 2A, and type 2X fibers.

➲   The main functional difference between the fiber types is the speed at which the fibers contract and relax, type 1 being the slow fibers and type 2 being the fast fibers.

➲   Although muscle fiber type is largely genetically determined, fibers are highly plastic and can adapt metabolically and functionally to different stimuli, such as specific exercise regimens.

➲   The information in the DNA of the nuclei is used to build new proteins in a process that involves transcription and translation.

CHAPTER 02

MUSCLE CONTRACTION AND ENERGY METABOLISM

The sliding filament theory describes our general understanding of how muscle contraction occurs. Specifically, the contractile filaments myosin and actin slide over each other, causing shortening of the sarcomeres. When muscle activation is sufficiently strong, this causes the entire muscle to shorten and mechanical force to be generated. Skeletal muscles are activated and controlled by the nervous system, and sufficient calcium and ATP must be present within the muscle fiber for muscle contraction to function. Skeletal muscle contractile activity accounts for a large portion of the body's ATP consumption, especially during physical activity. The ATP used for contractions is generated by the continuous breakdown of energy substrates. This chapter describes skeletal muscle energy metabolism, the neural control of muscle activity, and the cellular events that lead to muscle contraction.

FUEL FOR EXERCISE

Energy metabolism involves chemical processes that result in the production (synthesis) of molecules (anabolic reactions) or the breakdown of molecules (catabolic reactions). Energy is derived from nutrients and converted into biologically usable energy for muscle work. The human body is composed of up to 95% of four elements: oxygen, carbon, hydrogen, and nitrogen. Other elements present in small amounts include sodium, iron, zinc, potassium, magnesium, and calcium.

ATP (adenosine triphosphate) is the direct source of energy used by various tissue cells. An ATP molecule consists of an adenine part as the "backbone," a ribose part, and three individual phosphates linked together by high-energy bonds. When an ATPase enzyme cleaves one of these bonds, the energy is released in the following reaction: ATP → ADP + Pi + energy. This energy is used by myosin to interact with actin during muscle contraction. ATP is also used in the ion pumps of cells, which have the task of restoring the resting membrane potential of nerve and muscle cells. ATP is made from chemical energy in the form of fat, carbohydrates, and proteins that we consume with food.

Carbohydrates are composed of carbon, hydrogen, and oxygen. Carbohydrates stored in the body provide readily available energy, with 1 gram of carbohydrate producing about 4 kcal of energy. Carbohydrates are stored as glucose chains (glycogen) in the liver and other cells, but the largest stores are in skeletal muscle (about 500 g). Liver glycogen is used to supply glucose to the blood, while muscle glycogen provides immediate access to glucose in muscle fibers during intense work. Glycogen stored in muscle cannot leave the muscle cell, so muscle glycogen can only supply energy to skeletal muscle and not to other tissues. However, when glycogen is broken down, lactate is formed, which can be transported out of the muscle fibers and be used by other tissues as an energy substrate.

Fats are the largest energy reserve and are stored as triglycerides, which consist of a glycerol backbone and three individual fatty acids. Fat contains the same chemical elements as carbohydrates, but the amount of carbon relative to oxygen is much greater in fat than in carbohydrates. Stored fat is a good fuel source for prolonged physical activity because fat molecules contain high amounts of energy per unit weight (9 kcal per gram of fat).

While fat is primarily stored in adipose tissue, it is also found in other tissues, including skeletal muscle. Fat is transported in the body in the form of fatty acids, which are primarily burned in muscle fibers. Fatty acids are made up of long chains of carbon atoms joined at the ends with carboxyl groups (a carboxyl group consists of carbon, oxygen, and a hydrogen group).

Protein is the structural basis for all tissues and organs. The specific protein composition determines the appearance of the tissue and, to a large extent, its function. Proteins and amino acids serve as precursors to many hormones and neurotransmitters in the body. Proteins consist of long chains of amino acids held together by peptide bonds. In addition to carbon, hydrogen, and oxygen, amino acids also contain nitrogen.

The body can form various tissues, enzymes, and blood proteins from 20 different amino acids. The nine **essential amino acids** cannot be synthesized by the body and must therefore be obtained from the diet:

- Histidine
- Isoleucine
- Leucine
- Methionine
- Phenylalanine
- Threonine
- Tryptophan
- Valine
- Lysine

Skeletal muscle contains all amino acids. However, a large proportion (about 20%) consists of the branched-chain amino acids (BCAAs) leucine, valine, and isoleucine. Specific amino acid transporters can transport amino acids between the muscle and the blood.

Proteins contribute only slightly to ATP production in healthy people. However, the constituent amino acids are important metabolic intermediates in energy metabolism, and the amino acid alanine can be converted to glucose in the liver if needed. As a potential fuel source, protein contains about 4 kcal per gram. To be used as an energy substrate, protein must be broken down into the available amino acids.

Anaerobic ATP production

The metabolic pathways that produce ATP are classified as anaerobic if they do not involve oxygen and aerobic if they use oxygen in the mitochondria during ATP production. Both anaerobic and aerobic processes can be active simultaneously. The phosphocreatine system (PCr) is the fastest way to produce ATP because it involves only one reaction: ADP + PCr → ATP + Cr. The reaction catalyzed by the enzyme creatine kinase can generate ATP very quickly, but the stores only last for about 10 seconds of maximum work.

Glycolysis is the conversion of glucose into 2 molecules of pyruvate or lactate. Glucose stored as glycogen is first released by the enzyme glycogen phosphorylase, and a series of other enzyme reactions convert the energy bonds to glucose to eventually combine ADP + Pi to form ATP (Fig. 2.1). From glucose, the final products are 2 molecules of pyruvate or lactate, 2 ATPs, and 2 NADHs, which act as electron carriers in glycolysis. If glycogen is used as the starting substrate instead of glucose, the net production is 3 ATP.

Glycolysis releases hydrogen ions that must be buffered to avoid acidosis. Pyruvate and hydrogen ions can enter the mitochondria and contribute to oxidative ATP production during less intense muscle work. When energy demands are high, the rate of glycolysis is high, and in this case, the pyruvate takes up hydrogen to form lactate, which is then distributed through the blood inside and outside the muscle fiber. High levels of lactate in the blood indicate a high rate of energy conversion and are often used as a marker of fatigue.

Anaerobic metabolic pathways are the main suppliers of ATP during short bouts of intense work, such as a set of heavy resistance training. The limitation of anaerobic processes is the limited supply and accumulation of metabolites (e.g., inorganic phosphate groups) that are thought to contribute to muscle fatigue (see Chapter 13).

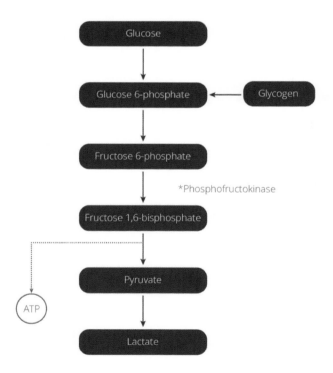

Figure 2.1.
Overview of anaerobic turnover of carbohydrates (glucose and glycogen) in glycolysis. The figure is simplified and does not show all the chemical reactions involved. *Phosphofructokinase is the enzyme considered rate–limiting in glycolysis.

Aerobic ATP production

During prolonged, moderate–intensity exercise, aerobic processes alone can supply muscles with ATP. However, the limitation of aerobic systems is that the rate of ATP production is slow. A comparison of the capacity of the aerobic and anaerobic energy systems is shown in Table 2.1.

Table 2.1.
Capacity vs. Power of the three major energy systems operative in resistance training. The table is adapted from the book Exercise Physiology: Human Bioenergetics and Its Applications (4th edition). George A. Brooks, Thomas D. Fahey and Kenneth Baldwin. McGraw–Hill Publishing Company, 2005.

	POWER (KCAL / MIN)	CAPACITY (KCAL TOTAL)
Instant sources (ATP + creatine phosphate)	36	11
Anaerobic breakdown of glycogen	16	15
Aerobic conversion of glycogen	10	2000

Aerobic energy metabolism takes place in the mitochondria of cells. Two major chemical pathways are involved in aerobic energy metabolism: the Krebs cycle (also called the citric acid cycle) and the electron transport chain (also called the respiratory chain). Pyruvate (from carbohydrates) and fatty acids (from fat) are broken down to acetyl–CoA. Hydrogen is then removed in the Krebs cycle, where the electron can be considered the high–energy component. The electrons then travel along the electron transport chain in a series of oxidation and reduction reactions. This electron transport provides a form of energy potential strong enough to combine ADP and Pi to form ATP, where the energy is now stored and can be used for muscle contraction. Oxygen (supplied to skeletal muscle via the cardiovascular system) accepts electrons in the final phase and water is formed.

Oxygen consumption is proportional to exercise intensity. At rest, oxygen uptake in a typical adult is about 300 ml per minute (3.5 ml/kg body weight per minute). When the whole body is working at a high intensity (e.g., running 1500 m), maximum oxygen uptake is reached. The maximum oxygen uptake can be up to 20 times higher than resting values in well–trained endurance athletes.

When pyruvate is converted to acetyl–CoA for aerobic metabolism, the net ATP number is 33. When glucose enters glycolysis directly, a net of 32 ATP is produced. Aerobic cellular respiration is about 34% effective in producing ATP and the remaining 66% forms thermal energy. Figure 2.2 illustrates the aerobic energy systems.

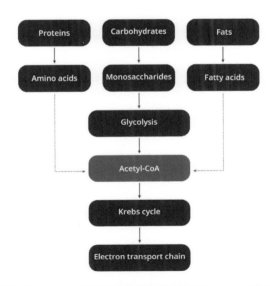

Figure 2.2.
Overview of the aerobic energy metabolism of fats, carbohydrates, and proteins.

Interaction between energy systems

Both the intensity and duration of work affect substrate use and determine which energy system predominates during exercise. In general, the ATP–phosphocreatine system is responsible for almost all energy production during high–intensity work lasting 1–5 seconds. For high–intensity work lasting longer than 5 seconds, the contribution of glycolysis increases significantly. This occurs gradually as the systems work in parallel and overlap. After more than 20 seconds of maximal work, glycolysis is the dominant process. For work periods longer than 45 seconds, a combination of all three systems is used. For work that lasts 60 seconds, the distribution is about 70–30% in favor of the anaerobic systems. For workouts that last two minutes, the distribution between anaerobic and aerobic processes is about 50–50%.

However, the intensity and duration of the workout are not the only factors that determine fuel selection. Training status and food intake can also be of great importance. Trained individuals can use fat as fuel to a greater extent than untrained individuals as intensity increases. A high carbohydrate intake ensures that the glycogen stores in the muscles are maximally filled, making it possible to use muscle glycogen as fuel for a longer period than if the diet were high in fat but low in carbohydrates.

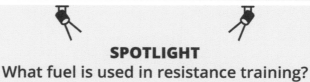

SPOTLIGHT
What fuel is used in resistance training?
· ·

The acute metabolic stress that occurs in muscles during resistance training is largely determined by the design of the training session. Generally, resistance training is performed at a high intensity while the volume of work is relatively low. Such a program stresses the anaerobic energy systems during the performance of each repetition. Both phosphocreatine and glycogen are therefore important energy substrates during a typical resistance training session. The extent to which the aerobic systems are stressed depends mainly on the duration of rest periods between sets and exercises. Resistance training in the form of circuit training with short rest periods can be very taxing on the aerobic systems and can therefore also lead to a metabolic response similar to traditional endurance training. Chapter 8 discusses the metabolic response and associated adaptations to resistance training in more detail.

NEUROMUSCULAR CONTROL OF MOVEMENT

The control of body movements is complex and requires integration and cooperation between the central nervous system (CNS) and the peripheral nervous system (PNS). The CNS includes the brain and spinal cord, while the PNS includes all neurons outside the CNS. The PNS is further divided into the somatic nervous system and the autonomic nervous system. Sensory neurons transmit information along afferent nerve fibers from peripheral receptors to the CNS. Conversely, motor nerves, which are under voluntary control, conduct signals along efferent nerve fibers from the CNS to peripheral tissues such as muscle. The autonomic nervous system is divided into sympathetic and parasympathetic nerve fibers, which are associated with various internal organs, the intestines, and smooth muscles, e.g., blood vessels.

The role of the brain in motor control

The brain can be divided into three parts: the brain stem, the cerebrum, and the cerebellum. These parts are all involved in the control of movement and therefore affect motor function and performance in resistance training. The brainstem is located at the base of the skull, above the spinal cord. The brainstem is responsible for many metabolic functions, cardiorespiratory control, and some complex reflexes. In the brainstem, neurons receive and integrate information from all regions of the CNS and work with higher functions to control muscle activity.

In addition, there are neural circuits responsible for controlling eye movements, muscle tone, balance, resistance to gravity, and many reflexes. One of the most important functions of the brainstem in controlling movement is maintaining postural tone. To accomplish this, the brainstem receives a large amount of sensory input from the body.

The cerebrum is a large part of the brain that is divided into the left and right hemispheres. The outer layer of the cerebrum is called the cerebral cortex and is made up of millions of neurons. The cerebral cortex performs three important motor functions:

- ➲ Organizes complex movements
- ➲ Stores learned experiences
- ➲ Receives sensory information

The part of the cerebral cortex primarily responsible for voluntary movements is the motor cortex. The motor cortex controls movements after input from subcortical parts (including the cerebellum). Thus, the motor cortex is the final point of contact where all inputs are summed and form the basis for the movement plan that is sent to the spinal cord.

The cerebellum has an important function in coordinating and monitoring complex movements. This work is done through connections to the motor cortex, brainstem, and spinal cord. One of the main tasks of the cerebellum is to fine–tune movements in response to feedback from receptors in tissues and joints (proprioceptors).

Initiation of movement begins with a rough sketch of the planned movement in the motivating areas of the brain (Fig. 2.3). The plan is transmitted to the cerebellum and basal nuclei, where it is transformed into more precise motor programs. These motor programs are sent via the thalamus to the motor cortex, where they are integrated with the help of the cerebellum. The integrated motor command is transmitted from the motor cortex to the spinal cord nerves in the PNS. Some modifications in response to afferent sensory feedback (e.g., pain) are still possible along this command line.

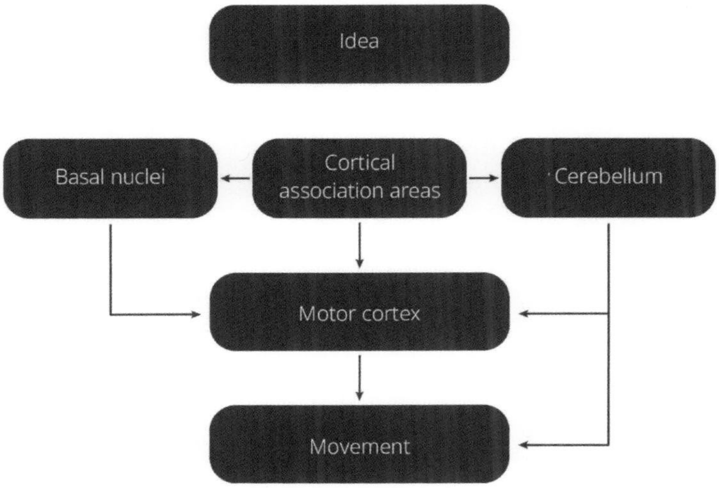

Figure 2.3.
Motor control of voluntary movements involves planning, initiation, and execution.

The anatomy of the motor nerves

Alpha motor neurons (Fig. 2.4) transmit efferent nerve signals to skeletal muscle fibers. These signals can range from a few millimeters to over 1 meter in length. The cell bodies of motor neurons are located in the spinal cord and contain the nucleus and organelles necessary to maintain neuron function. Special receptors called dendrites receive excitatory or inhibitory signals. A single axon (nerve fiber) extends from the cell body to the target tissue. A nerve is a bundle of many axons. Specialized Schwann cells surround the axon and form myelin sheaths that speed signal transmission. Regular gaps between these sheaths, called nodes of Ranvier, allow ion exchange during the transmission of nerve impulses. The axon divides into branches at the target muscle (the neuromuscular junction), and each skeletal muscle fiber is connected to the nerve cell via these branches.

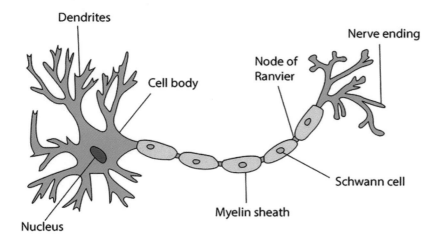

Figure 2.4.
The structure of the motor neuron. Revised from Dhp1080. The complete reference can be found in the Figure references section at the end of the book.

The action potential

The resting membrane potential of a motor neuron is negative, about –70 mV, because it contains more negatively charged ions (anions) inside than positively charged ions (cations). Sodium (Na^+), potassium (K^+), chloride (Cl^-), and calcium (Ca^{2+}) are important ions that maintain this negative membrane potential.

In the resting state, the inside of the cell contains very low concentrations of Na^+, Cl^-, and Ca^{2+}, but a high concentration of K^+. The outside of the cell contains higher concentrations of Na^+, Cl^-, and Ca^{2+}, but lower concentrations of K^+. Ions are exchanged in large amounts only when voltage–sensitive channels are open. The ion exchange that takes place is regulated by the sodium–potassium pump, an energy–consuming ion pump that ensures that the negative membrane potential is maintained.

When a stimulatory (excitatory) signal arriving at the dendrites is strong enough, it causes Na^+ channels to open and Na^+ to diffuse into the cell. This depolarization alters the local membrane potential, making it more positive (Fig. 2.5). When the threshold is reached, an action potential (nerve impulse) is triggered. The action potential propagates distally along the axon and adjacent Na^+ channels open in sequence. Shortly after the Na^+ channels open, the K^+ channels also open, allowing K^+ to flow out of the cell along the concentration gradient. The Na^+ channels are closed, and the membrane potential is repolarized, while the interior of the cell returns to the negative state.

Once an action potential is initiated, it is propagated along the axon to the nerve terminal, with no voltage lost along the way. This is called the *all–or–nothing principle*. The speed of an action potential is about 50 m/s, and it is generally possible to trigger action potentials about 5–30 times per second.

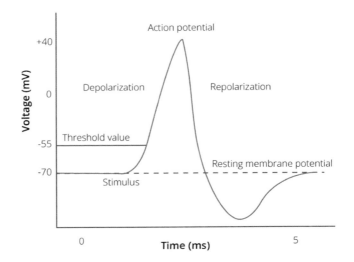

Figure 2.5.
Action potential overview. When a stimulus alters the membrane potential beyond the critical threshold, there is a rapid depolarization followed by repolarization.

Motor units

A motor unit consists of a single motor neuron and all the muscle fibers innervated by that neuron (Fig. 2.6). The number of muscle fibers innervated by a single motor neuron is called the innervation ratio. This ratio varies greatly within and between different muscles. In the large muscles of the leg, there are typically hundreds to thousands of fibers per motor neuron, whereas in the smaller fine motor muscles, there are a much smaller number of fibers associated with each neuron.

The muscle fibers of a single motor unit are generally of the same type. When a motor neuron gives an action potential, all the fibers belonging to that motor unit are stimulated to contract. A motor unit can therefore be considered the smallest functional unit in the neuromuscular system. The fibers in a motor unit are rarely adjacent to each other. Instead, they are distributed in the large extremities over areas about 5–10 mm deep. A muscle cross–section of about 10 mm may contain fibers belonging to twenty individual motor units. This allows the muscle to distribute force evenly over relatively large areas throughout the muscle when the motor units are recruited.

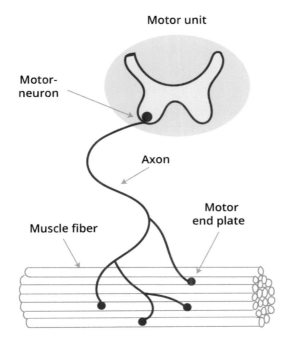

Motor unit

Motor-neuron

Axon

Muscle fiber

Motor end plate

Figure 2.6.
Motor unit. A motor neuron and the muscle fibers innervated by the neuron are called a motor unit. Motor neurons are located in the anterior part of the spinal cord.

The incredible range of body movements that can be performed is made possible by the organized activation of different groups of motor units. This is accomplished in two ways. The first way to control muscle strength is to change the number of motor units recruited. This is called **recruitment strategy.** When only a low force is required, very few motor units are recruited. However, when a high force is required, many units are recruited to activate more muscle fibers.

The second strategy is to change the firing rate (discharge rate) of the action potentials. This is called **rate coding**. Both strategies are often used to regulate the force.

The force that can be produced by a motor unit is directly proportional to the ratio of innervation, with more fibers thus producing greater muscle force. The voluntary recruitment of motor units is controlled by the central nervous system. A high voluntary effort leads to a strong neural drive and more motor units reach their activation threshold. **The size principle** describes the highly organized recruitment of motor units ranging in size from the smallest to the largest (Fig. 2.7). The smallest motor units are recruited first because they have a low firing threshold. These units innervate type 1 fibers. When higher forces are required, larger motor units are gradually recruited. Maximal forces require maximal effort to recruit as many fibers as possible. The largest motor units innervate the fastest type 2 fibers.

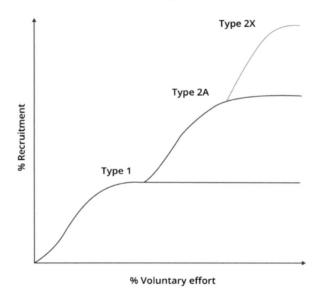

% Voluntary effort

Figure 2.7.
The size principle. With increasing physical strain and exertion, the recruitment of the motor units increases in an orderly manner, from the smallest units to the largest.

The neuromuscular junction

Each individual muscle fiber is connected to the nervous system by a single nerve branch. The point where the nerve branch meets the muscle fiber is called the **neuromuscular junction.** However, the motor nerve does not make physical contact with the muscle fiber. Instead, a synaptic cleft forms between the nerve terminal and the postsynaptic membrane of the muscle fiber. An action potential arriving at the nerve ending increases the permeability of the nerve to calcium. Calcium stimulation causes the neurotransmitter acetylcholine, which is found in vesicles at the nerve terminal, to be released into the synaptic cleft. Acetylcholine diffuses through the cleft and attaches to acetylcholine receptors on the postsynaptic membrane (Fig. 2.8).

Just like nerves, muscle fibers can also be depolarized. The negative resting membrane potential is maintained similarly to a nerve by regulating ion concentrations. The binding of acetylcholine to its receptor at the endplate increases Na^+ permeability and depolarizes the muscle fiber. The resulting endplate potential propagates along the muscle fibers even though the muscle fibers are not myelinated. In this way, the nerve signals that started in the brain can eventually trigger muscle contractions. The action potential of the muscle fibers propagates along the T–tubules, which are located deep within the fibers. This triggers the release of calcium from the sarcoplasmic reticulum, the specialized organelle that stores calcium in the muscle fiber. The calcium released into the sarcoplasm binds to troponin to initiate the cross–bridge cycle that leads to muscle contraction.

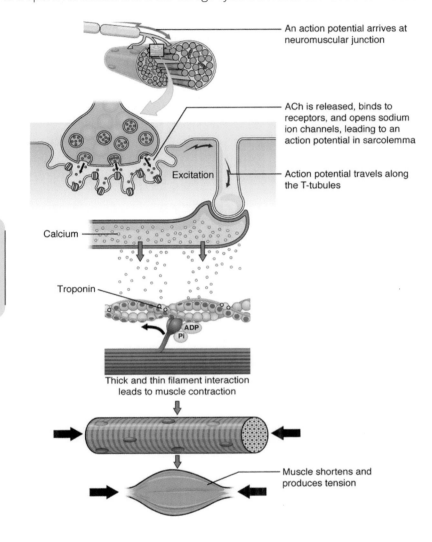

An action potential arrives at neuromuscular junction

ACh is released, binds to receptors, and opens sodium ion channels, leading to an action potential in sarcolemma

Action potential travels along the T-tubules

Excitation

Calcium

Troponin

ADP
Pi

Thick and thin filament interaction leads to muscle contraction

Muscle shortens and produces tension

Figure 2.8.
The neuromuscular junction and muscle contraction. Created by OpenStax. The complete reference can be found in the Figure references section at the end of the book.

MUSCLE CONTRACTION: THE SLIDING FILAMENT THEORY

Muscle contraction occurs by shortening of the myofibrils as the contractile proteins "slide" over each other via cross–bridges, with the myosin heads forming strong bonds with the actin filaments and then pulling the actin over the myosin molecules (Fig. 2.8). The term *excitation–contraction coupling* describes the sequence of events in which the nerve impulse reaches the muscle membrane and results in muscle shortening due to the cross–bridge activity between actin and myosin. The energy for the cross–bridge cycle comes from the breakdown of ATP by the enzyme ATPase, which is located on the myosin head. The breakdown of ATP to ADP and a free phosphate ion (Pi) provides energy for the cross–bridges so that the actin filaments are pulled across the myosin. The contraction cycle must be repeated over and over to achieve complete shortening of the muscle.

The first step in muscular contraction is when the nerve impulse released in the brain reaches the neuromuscular junction, as described in the previous section. Depolarization is conducted through the transverse tubules (T-tubules) deep into the muscle fiber. When the action potential is near the sarcoplasmic reticulum, calcium is released and diffuses into the muscle to bind to troponin. The calcium allows myosin to bind to actin because binding to troponin causes the tropomyosin protein covering the binding sites on actin to move, exposing the binding sites. As long as action potentials arrive at the neuromuscular junction, there is enough calcium in the sarcoplasm to ensure that muscle contraction can continue (at least until the muscle is exhausted).

When action potentials stop arriving, usually because we intentionally interrupt our work, calcium is rapidly pumped back into the sarcoplasmic reticulum in a process that requires ATP. Tropomyosin then covers the myosin binding site on actin, preventing the formation of new strong cross-bridges. However, when calcium is present, strong bonds between myosin and actin can be formed. The strong cross-bridge initiates a release of the energy stored in the myosin molecule. This results in an angular movement of each cross-bridge, causing the muscle to shorten. When new ATP attaches to the myosin head, the strong bond breaks, and a weak bond is formed. The enzyme ATPase breaks down the ATP bound to the myosin, and the cross-bridge cycle continues. As long as free calcium is available to bind to troponin and ATP can be degraded, contraction continues.

SUMMARY

- ⮂ ATP is the direct source of energy for cells. ATP is produced by the breakdown of carbohydrates, fats, and proteins.

- ⮂ When an ATPase enzyme cleaves the ATP molecule, energy is released for muscle work.

- ⮂ Carbohydrates provide readily available energy, with 1 gram of carbohydrate providing about 4 kcal of energy.

- ⮂ Carbohydrates are stored as glucose chains (glycogen) in the liver and other cells, but the largest stores are in skeletal muscle.

- ⮂ Fats (9 kcal per gram) are the largest energy reserve and are stored as triglycerides mainly in adipose tissue.

- ⮂ Protein is the structural basis for all tissues and organs and is not a primary energy substrate for muscle work.

- ⮂ Proteins consist of long chains of amino acids held together by peptide bonds.

- ⮂ The metabolic pathways that produce ATP are classified as anaerobic if they do not involve oxygen in ATP production and aerobic if they use oxygen in the mitochondria.

- ⮂ The phosphocreatine system (PCr) is the fastest metabolic pathway to produce ATP: ADP + PCr → ATP + Cr.

- ⮂ Anaerobic glycolysis involves the conversion of glucose or glycogen to pyruvate or lactate.

- ⮂ Two major chemical pathways are involved in aerobic energy metabolism: the Krebs cycle and the electron transport chain.

- ⮂ Carbohydrates, fats, and proteins can be used in aerobic energy production and generate ATP using oxygen.

- ⮂ The intensity and duration of exercise are the main factors in substrate selection and the metabolic pathway during exercise.

- ⮂ Our body movements are controlled by the central nervous system (CNS) and the peripheral nervous system (PNS).

- The part of the brain primarily responsible for voluntary movements is the motor cortex.

- The peripheral motor nervous system originates in the spinal cord, where alpha motor neurons send nerve signals (action potentials) to skeletal muscle fibers.

- A motor unit consists of a single motor neuron and all the muscle fibers innervated by that neuron.

- Muscle strength is regulated mainly by changing the number of motor units recruited (recruitment strategy) or by changing the firing frequency at which the motor units send action potentials (rate coding).

- The size principle describes a highly organized strategy for recruiting motor units in order of size, from the smallest units (innervating slow fibers) to the largest units (innervating fast fibers).

- The point where the nerve branch meets the muscle fiber is called the neuromuscular junction.

- The action potential of the muscle fibers propagates along the T–tubules, which are located deep within the fibers. This triggers the release of calcium from the sarcoplasmic reticulum, a large, specialized organelle that stores calcium and surrounds the muscle fiber.

- Muscle contraction occurs through myofibril shortening, in which contractile proteins "slide" over each other using cross–bridges, with myosin heads forming strong bonds with actin filaments and then pulling the actin over the myosin molecules.

- The energy for the cross–bridge cycle comes from the breakdown of ATP.

- When ATP attaches to the myosin head, the strong bond between myosin and actin breaks and a weak bond is formed. The enzyme ATPase in turn breaks down ATP bound to myosin. As long as action potentials reach the fiber and free calcium is available to bind to troponin, the contraction continues.

03

CHAPTER 03

BIOLOGICAL BASIS OF FORCE PRODUCTION

The force generated in a joint is usually the result of several separate forces generated by muscles working together. For example, during a normal knee extension, all four quadriceps muscles are active. At the same time, the synergist muscles help stabilize the joint. While the coordinated motor commands sent to agonists, synergists, and antagonists are important for net force production, the maximum force that can be produced in a joint is also proportional to the physiological cross-sectional area of the agonist muscle, as this represents the number of parallel sarcomeres that actively transmit force to the tendon. Simply put, a larger muscle is usually a stronger muscle. However, the relationship between strength and muscle size is not perfect, as other factors also influence force production. The importance of the nervous system has already been mentioned, but other factors such as fiber types, anatomy, biomechanics, pennation angle, fascicle length, and extracellular matrix composition can also influence the ability to develop force. This chapter provides an overview of the most important factors that determine the force development of skeletal muscle.

NERVOUS SYSTEM CONTROL

Twitches, summation, and tetanus

When a single action potential triggers the release of calcium from the sarcoplasmic reticulum, it induces a brief muscle "twitch" that produces only minimal shortening of the muscle. A twitch has a very short latency period, lasting only a few milliseconds, followed by a shortening phase (contraction) that lasts about 40 milliseconds. This is followed by relaxation, which lasts about 50 milliseconds. The timing of these phases depends on the fiber types, with slow type 1 fibers contracting and relaxing slowly and fast type 2 fibers having faster shortening and relaxation times due to faster calcium release and higher myosin ATPase activity. If a second action potential occurs before the muscle is fully relaxed, additional calcium is released and the resulting force adds to the first twitch in a process called summation (Fig. 3.1).

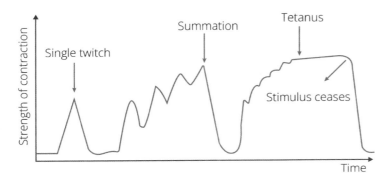

Figure 3.1.
Schematic illustration of a single twitch, summation, and tetanic contraction.

Summation continues with increasing firing frequency until a point is reached where no further summation is possible (usually at 30–50 Hz), which is called a tetanic contraction. The muscle actions performed during whole–body movements are the result of summed contractions. Higher firing frequencies are associated with progressively increasing force development. However, there are factors that complicate this principle. First, firing frequency varies widely between different types of motor neurons, ranging from about 5 to 30 Hz, and the large motor units innervating type 2 fibers may emit action potentials much more frequently than small motor neurons.

Second, the contractile properties of muscle fibers differ, with slow fibers contracting and relaxing more slowly than fast fibers, allowing more time for summation. Third, different muscle groups have different control methods and principles for neural activation. For example, force in the hand muscles can be increased by activating more motor units in sequence while simultaneously increasing the firing frequency. In contrast, the force produced in the quadriceps muscle depends largely on the proportion of motor units recruited, because the firing frequency varies relatively little, at least for contractions up to about 80% of the maximum force [16]. Finally, a muscle produces a higher force in response to a single twitch or brief stimulation if it has been active recently. This phenomenon is called ***post–activation potentiation*** (see Chapter 5).

Proprioceptors

Specialized sensory receptors, the proprioceptors, are located in joints and tissues. These receptors respond to changes in muscle length, joint angle, chemical environment, pain, pressure, and tension. The most common proprioceptors are free nerve endings, Golgi tendon organs, and muscle spindles. These proprioceptors provide constant feedback to the CNS and can alter the body's motor commands. They can also influence the circulatory response to movement and potentially contribute to fatigue via central command mechanisms (fatigue is discussed in more detail in Chapter 13).

The Golgi organs are located in the tendons and provide continuous information to the CNS about the tension generated by the contracting muscles exerted on the tendon. Increased tension increases the excitation of the Golgi tendon organs, and this information is relayed to the CNS via sensory neurons to trigger inhibitory signals, if necessary, to limit further activation of the muscles. This reflex provides a safety mechanism that protects the body from excessive muscle contractions.

The muscle spindles are collections of specialized, thin muscle cells distributed along the contracting muscle fibers. Their main function is to provide continuous information about muscle length to the CNS. This is done via primary sensory nerve endings, which respond to changes in dynamic length, and secondary sensory nerve endings, which monitor static muscle length. Gamma motor neurons (as opposed to alpha motor neurons, which innervate skeletal muscle fibers) are connected to muscle spindles. The primary nerve terminals respond to rapid muscle lengthening by sending action potentials to the CNS in the spinal cord, where there is a synaptic connection to the dendrites of the pool of alpha motor neurons. Thus, excitation of the primary sensory neurons can lead to excitation of the alpha motor neurons following rapid lengthening of the muscle. This leads to a contraction that interrupts the rapid muscle lengthening. This is called the stretch reflex, which can easily be triggered by a sharp tap on the patellar tendon (knee–jerk reflex).

MUSCLE ACTIONS

One of the most obvious factors affecting force development is the type of muscle action. The different muscle actions can be divided into isometric and dynamic actions. In isometric (static) muscle actions, there is no change in muscle length. Dynamic movements can be further divided into concentric and eccentric muscle actions (Fig. 3.2). In concentric muscle actions, the muscle is shortened (origin and insertion approach each other). In eccentric actions, the muscle contraction occurs while the muscle lengthens. Eccentric actions therefore occur when an external force is controlled in a coordinated way, for example when we lower a weight, land from a jump or decelerate and change direction.

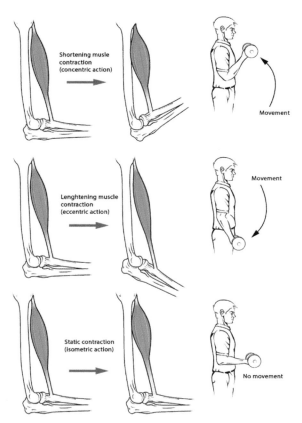

Figure 3.2.
Concentric, eccentric, and isometric muscle actions. Created by OpenStax. The complete reference can be found in the Figure references section at the end of the book.

The mechanisms of force generation differ between concentric and eccentric actions. This explains why force generation in eccentric actions can exceed the force of concentric actions, even though concentric actions require 4–6 times more energy. Thus, much less ATP is required for the cross–bridge cycle in negative lengthening actions than in shortening concentric actions, in which myosin must actively pull on actin to cause shortening of the sarcomere.

Concentric and eccentric actions also differ in their strategy of neuronal activation. Neural activation is significantly greater in concentric actions than in eccentric actions. Therefore, the neural drive is lower in eccentric actions, which is due to both lower recruitment of motor units and lower firing frequency. It is thought that feedback from various proprioceptors, decreased activity of the motor cortex, and some form of presynaptic inhibition all contribute to this phenomenon of neuronal inhibition during eccentric movements [17].

The successive combination of eccentric and concentric actions, as in running and jumping, is called the stretch–shortening cycle. Muscle strength generally increases during movements that involve the stretch–shortening cycle. Although the underlying mechanisms of this effect are still debated, the general explanation is that both the contractile and elastic elements in the muscles are enhanced.

SPOTLIGHT
Why can muscle produce more force eccentrically than concentrically?
· · · · · · · · · · · · · · · · · · · ·

Remember that force depends on the number of active cross–bridges (myosin and actin that are tightly bound together). Concentric actions can generate less force because myosin and actin have less time to form strong cross bridges. The high demand for shortening means that the myosin heads must change their position on the actin filaments to accomplish the shortening. In addition, the so–called S2 complex on the myosin molecule is not fully extended during rapid shortening contractions, which decreases the force between myosin and actin [17]. During isometric and eccentric muscle actions, myosin and actin have enough time to form strong cross–bridges. In addition, the large protein titin acts like a spring that can store and then release elastic energy. It also appears that titin can interact with actin and actively contribute to force generation during eccentric movements [18].

MUSCLE ARCHITECTURE

The architecture of the muscle affects its ability to generate force. Physiological cross–sectional area, pennation angle, and fiber length, as well as the distribution of fiber types, are all factors that have an influence on muscle force and shortening velocity. Maximum force development is proportional to the number of parallel sarcomeres, while maximum shortening velocity correlates with the number of sarcomeres in series and thus fiber and fascicle length.

A typical fascicle length in the thigh and calf muscles is 5–10 cm. The fascicles are relatively short because the direction of the fibers is usually angled in relation to the line of origin and insertion. Examples include the vastus muscles of the thigh, which face the deeper connective tissue membrane (aponeurosis) at an angle of about 10–20°. The disadvantage of such a fiber arrangement is that some of the force generated disappears before being transmitted to the tendon insertion. This loss of force is proportional to the cosine of the pennation angle, so the greater the pennation angle, the less the force in the longitudinal/anatomical direction of the muscle. However, the advantage is that more muscle fibers can be accommodated within the same anatomical cross–section of the muscle (Fig. 3.3). The resulting larger physiological cross–sectional area provides greater potential for force development. The theoretical advantage of pennate muscles in terms of force development is at an angle of approximately 45 degrees. The effect of resistance training on muscle architecture is discussed in more detail in Chapter 9.

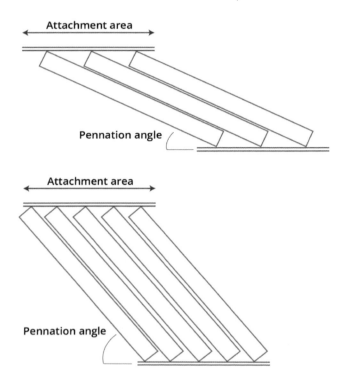

Figure 3.3.
Schematic representation of the pennation angle in skeletal muscle. A larger pennation angle means that more contractile units can be packed into the same anatomical length (referred to as the attachment area in the figure), resulting in a larger physiological cross–sectional area of the muscle.

THE CONTRACTILE PROPERTIES OF THE MUSCLE FIBERS

The contractile properties of skeletal muscle fibers were briefly mentioned in Chapter 1. The three main contractile properties that are important for force development in different situations are:

- ➲ Maximum force generation
- ➲ Shortening velocity
- ➲ Efficiency

The maximum force output of fibers is usually expressed as force per cross–sectional area (specific tension or specific force). The rate of contraction is the maximum rate of shortening of individual fibers and is referred to as Vmax. Factors that determine Vmax include fiber type, calcium release, and myosin ATPase activity. Fast fibers can produce force faster than slow fibers due to higher ATPase activity and faster calcium release. Thus, fast fibers have a higher shortening velocity and thus a significantly higher maximum power development than slow type 1 fibers. For a given contractile force output of a muscle, the velocity in a muscle with a higher proportion of fast fibers is always greater.

Finally, the efficiency of a muscle fiber is important for its ability to sustain a given force over a long period of time. An efficient fiber requires less energy (ATP per given work output) than a less efficient fiber. Type 1 slow fibers are more efficient than fast fibers.

MECHANICAL RELATIONSHIPS

The force–length relationship

The length at which the muscle works affects the force development in a joint. This relationship is called the force–length or length–tension relationship and can be demonstrated at the level of sarcomeres or in isolated fibers, where fiber tension is measured at different portions of the fiber length (Fig. 3.4). Such experiments show that the optimal sarcomere length, which produces the best overlap between myosin and actin and thus the greatest force, is at about 110–120% of the resting muscle length.

At the level of the whole muscle, muscle length is determined primarily by joint angle. For the quadriceps muscle group, optimal muscle length is achieved at a knee angle of about 120° (60° from full extension). Deviations from this angle reduce the strength to varying degrees, depending on how much the muscle is shortened or lengthened.

The reason why less force is produced in a stretched or shortened muscle is related to the length of the sarcomere and the number of cross–bridges that can produce tension. Force production is hindered when the sarcomere length is short because the actin filaments partially overlap at the opposite end of the sarcomere. Lower force potential also results when the sarcomere extends beyond the optimal length, as this also reduces the overlap between actin and myosin filaments. At the optimal length, in principle, all myosin heads can bind to the actin filaments.

It is obvious that the muscle generates force at different joint angles during dynamic movements. It is also important to note that the force–length relationship varies depending on whether individual sarcomeres or a whole muscle with intact tendon and connective tissue are examined. When the muscle is stretched, the contribution of the elastic components to force production increases. Thus, a whole muscle can continue to produce a large force even if the sarcomeres are stretched beyond the point where the overlap between myosin and actin is optimal. Thus, considerable stretching of the muscle is required for force production to decrease.

Figure 3.4.
Muscle force–length relationship. See chapter text for further guidance.

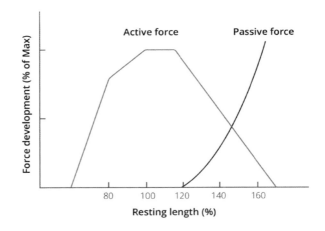

The force–velocity relationship

The so-called force–velocity relationship also determines the muscle's ability to generate force. In a concentric muscle action, force decreases as the speed of contraction increases (Fig. 3.5). This can be explained at the myofilament level by the fact that it takes time for the cross-bridges to work and produce a significant shortening effect with the power strokes. During an isometric contraction, where the velocity is zero, maximum force can be developed because many cross-bridges can be in a strong binding state at any given time. Equal or even higher forces are possible in eccentric muscle actions because the muscle is not shortened. Therefore, the cross-bridges can be in the strong binding position for a greater proportion of the time than during fast contractions. At the fiber level, it is noted that type 2 fibers produce higher forces than type 1 fibers for a given absolute velocity, but both types of fibers lose force with increasing velocity.

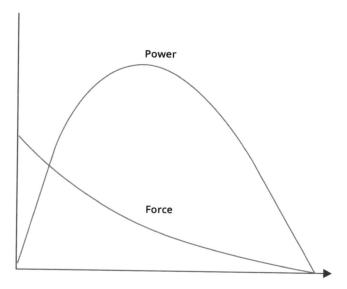

Figure 3.5.
The force–velocity relationship and power–velocity relationship of skeletal muscles. See chapter text for further guidance.

Power development

The power development of the muscle is determined by the interaction between force and velocity. Thus, mechanical power can be defined as work/time or force × velocity. Therefore, peak power occurs where the product of force and velocity is greatest (Fig. 3.5). Individual fibers tend to reach their peak power when the fiber is producing only about 20% of its maximum force. In isolated movements, such as seated knee extensions, peak power is usually reached at velocities equal to about 1/3 of the maximum contraction velocity. The speed or intensity at which peak power occurs in different types of strength exercises varies depending on the type of exercise, whether it is a multi-joint or single-joint exercise, etc. However, most often it occurs at a much higher load/force than in isolated experiments (i.e., at much higher forces than the 20% of maximum cited for individual fibers).

Type 2 fibers can produce higher power than type 1 fibers because the rate of shortening is higher in the faster fiber types. Peak power is therefore greater in fast muscle fibers. Power is important in many sporting contexts, but also for physical function in the elderly, as high muscle power reduces the risk of falls.

Biomechanics

There are several biomechanical factors that affect the muscle's ability to generate force, and these factors also interact with the mechanical relationships (force–length and force–velocity). One such important biomechanical factor is the lever arm. The torque (moment force) across a joint is determined by the applied load/resistance multiplied by the perpendicular lever distance from the fulcrum in the joint to the center of mass of the load. For a biceps curl, the torque in the elbow joint is greatest when the joint is flexed at about 90 degrees. At this angle, the greatest muscle force is required from the elbow flexors. The sticking point refers to the position within the range of motion of an exercise where the combination of lever arm and muscle length is least favorable. At this point, the execution of the lift becomes most difficult and is usually the point at which the exercise fails.

The internal moment arm, which is the distance between the tendon insertion to the bone and the pivot point in the joint, also plays a role in the biomechanics of force generation (Fig. 3.6). This tendon moment arm is genetically determined and can vary between different muscles and to some degree between different individuals. A long tendon moment arm is positive for the ability to develop high torque, while a short lever arm can instead cause a large change in joint angle for a given contraction. Thus, the length of the tendon moment arm plays a role in the ability to generate high force and high velocity.

Figure 3.6.
Biomechanics of lever arms and forces acting around a joint. The figure was created using BioRender.com with accompanying publishing license.

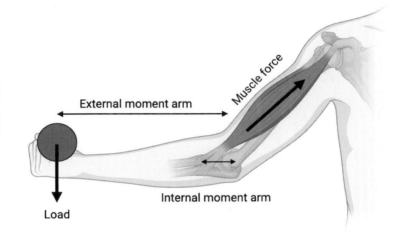

FORCE TRANSFER

The cytoskeletal network of muscle transmits force both within and between muscle fibers. In mice, an estimated 80% of the force is transmitted laterally from proteins within the fibers to extracellular proteins outside the fiber [19]. Key components of force transmission are intracellular proteins such as titin and dystrophin, the dystrophin–associated glycoprotein complex (DAGC), and integrins, as well as extracellular proteins that determine the properties of connective tissue and tendons (collagen proteins). Various experimental models in both animals and humans have shown that these proteins are essential for the transmission of force from muscle to bone. This is particularly important for the ability to generate force quickly, which is called the rate of force development.

Titin is an important protein for force transfer and general contractile function. Titin was discovered in the 1970s and was called "connectin" at the time [20]. Titin was therefore not included in the original sliding filament theory of Andrew Huxley in the 1950s. We now know that titin acts as an anchor between myosin filaments and Z–discs in sarcomeres. Titin becomes active during eccentric muscle movements and "folds" to store energy that can even match the mechanical energy generated by the ATP–dependent myosin and actin filaments. By influencing the functions of titin in mouse models, the importance of this protein for muscle function has been demonstrated [21]. An overview of the most important factors for the muscle's ability to develop force can be found in Figure 3.7.

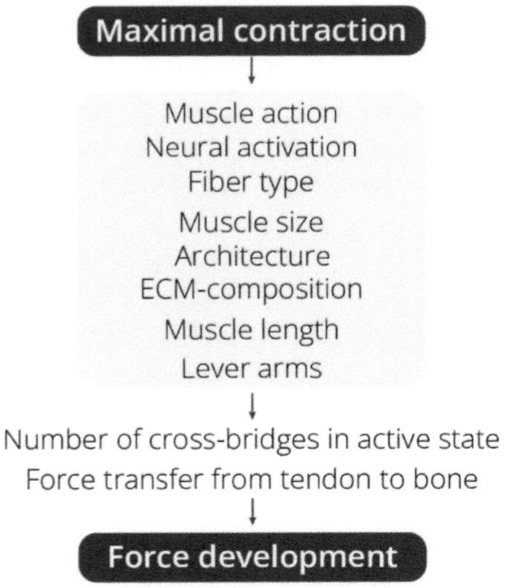

Maximal contraction

Muscle action
Neural activation
Fiber type

Muscle size
Architecture
ECM-composition

Muscle length
Lever arms

Number of cross-bridges in active state
Force transfer from tendon to bone

Force development

Figure 3.7.
Summary of the major factors that determine the development of muscle force during a maximal contraction.

SUMMARY

- In muscle actions performed during whole–body movements, single nerve impulses are summed into tetanic contractions.

- The firing frequency varies between different types of motor units.

- Sensory receptors, called proprioceptors, protect our muscles and joints by providing feedback to the central nervous system via sensory (afferent) nerve fibers.

- Golgi tendon organs are located in tendons and provide continuous information to the CNS about the tension generated by contracting muscles.

- The muscle spindles provide continuous information to the CNS about muscle length.

- Maximum force output is slightly greater in eccentric compared to concentric muscle actions.

- Concentric actions are more energy consuming and require greater neural activation for a given force output than eccentric actions.

- The sequential combination of eccentric and concentric actions is referred to as the stretch–shortening cycle.

- Physiological cross–sectional area and fiber length, along with the distribution of fiber types and the ability of the nervous system to activate the muscle, are the most important factors affecting force production and shortening velocity of skeletal muscles.

- The pennation angle of the fascicles affects force capacity, with a fiber direction in line with the origin and insertion favoring a high shortening velocity, while a more angled fiber direction increases the physiological cross–sectional area, providing greater potential for force production.

- The length at which the muscle works influences the force development across a joint. This relationship is referred to as the force–length relationship.

- During a concentric muscle action, force decreases as the rate of contraction increases, which is referred to as the force–velocity relationship.

⮌ The power output of the muscle is determined by the interaction between force and velocity, where mechanical power is defined as work/time or force × velocity.

⮌ There are several biomechanical factors that affect the muscle's ability to develop force, including the lever arm of the working muscle and the tendon moment arm.

⮌ A cytoskeletal network transmits force within and between muscle fibers to connective tissue and tendons, which in turn transmit force to the bone.

04

MUSCLE PROTEIN TURNOVER

The skeletal muscle is constantly remodeled by the processes of protein synthesis (in which amino acids are used to build new proteins) and protein degradation (in which proteins are broken down into amino acids). Over time, these dynamic processes control the quantity and quality of proteins in our bodies, including skeletal muscle. When muscle protein synthesis is greater than breakdown over a predictable period of time, there is an accumulation of muscle proteins and an increase in muscle mass (hypertrophy). In contrast, when protein breakdown is greater than protein synthesis, there is a net loss of muscle mass (atrophy). This chapter describes the protein turnover of skeletal muscle and discusses the effects of resistance training on these processes.

DYNAMIC SYNTHESIS AND DEGRADATION

Amino acids are constantly assembled into new proteins in the ribosomes of cells. Likewise, there is a constant breakdown of proteins into individual amino acids. Most amino acids are stored in the various tissues of the body. There is only a small circulating pool of amino acids, consisting mainly of recently digested amino acids. These amino acids are taken up by the tissues for the synthesis of new proteins. In this way, protein breakdown is directly linked to protein synthesis. Unlike fat and glycogen, there is no major storage site for protein. Excessive protein intake therefore leads to greater oxidation of amino acids along with increased nitrogen excretion.

Many structural proteins and enzymes have a high turnover rate. About 20% of the basic energy consumption is caused by protein metabolism in the body. The very short lifespan of some enzymes is important for the body to respond quickly to new conditions, such as different metabolic demands. Thus, there is a constant build-up and breakdown of muscle proteins, and these processes are regulated by complex molecular programs, which are described in more detail in Chapter 7.

The balance between synthesis (anabolism) and breakdown (catabolism) can be influenced by a variety of factors, with resistance training playing an important role. Even more dramatic effects occur in the case of infections or complete muscle disuse, in which a clear muscle degradation can be observed. Muscle atrophy is also common during extreme physical inactivity, aging, starvation, and several chronic diseases.

SPOTLIGHT
What happens to protein after a meal?
. . . .

When we eat a meal that contains 20 grams of protein, about 50% of that protein is absorbed and stored by the intestines and liver before the remaining amino acids reach the systemic circulation. The portion of amino acids that enter the bloodstream are mainly the branched-chain amino acids, as these are not broken down in the liver. Most of the amino acids that enter the circulation are used for energy metabolism or neurotransmitter production. This leaves about 10–20% (2–4 grams) of the original protein quantity, and this portion reaches the skeletal muscles and can contribute to the synthesis of new muscle proteins [22].

METHODS FOR MEASURING PROTEIN TURNOVER

Most knowledge about muscle protein turnover comes from studies that have examined mixed muscle protein turnover. This means that the turnover of all muscle proteins is examined, regardless of whether they are contractile, mitochondrial, or sarcoplasmic proteins. Myofibrillar proteins are by far the most abundant proteins, accounting for 70–85% of the total protein pool in muscle.

Skeletal muscle is a plastic tissue that breaks down and replaces 1–2% of its protein pool per day. This is a high turnover rate compared to, for example, bone tissue, where turnover averages about 10% per year. Recent research has studied protein metabolism in the brain (neocortex and hippocampus) and, surprisingly, protein synthesis was 3–4 times higher than in skeletal muscle [23]. Techniques for studying muscle protein turnover have been refined in recent decades, but there are still limitations, not least in estimating muscle protein breakdown.

Nitrogen balance

The nitrogen we take in with food comes from proteins. Nitrogen cannot be stored in the body but must be excreted in the urine. By measuring the nitrogen in food and the amount of nitrogen excreted by the body, the nitrogen balance can be calculated. If the nitrogen balance is positive, it means that the body stores more protein than it breaks down, and vice versa. Measurements of nitrogen balance at different protein intakes form the basis for the recommended daily protein intake for the population (0.8 g/kg body weight). However, in the context of resistance training, nitrogen balance is a very crude measure because it does not reflect the protein balance of the muscles. The muscle protein balance can be negative even if the total nitrogen balance of the body is positive. Thus, nitrogen balance only provides a general indication of whether the body is in an anabolic or catabolic state and does not provide information about skeletal muscle protein metabolism.

Tracers

A tracer is a substance that can be tracked in the body. To determine muscle protein synthesis, labeled amino acids or "amino acid tracers" are used. These amino acids have an extra neutron that allows them to be traced. By tracking what happens to these labeled amino acids, protein synthesis and degradation can be measured using repeated muscle biopsies. It is then possible to track the rate at which the labeled amino acids are incorporated into muscle proteins. This method provides a measure of **fractional synthetic rate** (FSR) expressed in %/hour. An FSR value of 0.04%/hour means that protein turnover is approximately 1–2% per day. This means that the entire muscle has been renewed in about 3 months.

While FSR is a measure of protein synthesis in muscle, it does not indicate the type of protein being synthesized. It may be contractile proteins as well as mitochondrial proteins or proteins in the cytoplasm. To determine this more accurately, different protein fractions can be isolated from the muscle sample. This allows a more specific measurement of protein synthesis, e.g., for myofibrillar proteins, the protein fraction most stimulated by resistance training.

Whereas resistance training in the untrained state leads to an increase in both myofibrillar and mitochondrial protein synthesis, after several weeks of training the increase occurs mainly in the myofibrillar fraction [24], indicating that the protein turnover response to acute resistance training becomes more specific with chronic training. In the initial phase, the response is general, and widespread effects of training can be expected. Over time, it becomes more difficult to achieve substantial adaptations, and they are increasingly directed toward meeting the precise requirements of the specific form of training.

Deuterium oxide (heavy water)

A more recent technique for studying protein synthesis is the use of deuterium oxide, also called heavy water. The main difference between this technique and the use of amino acid tracers is that protein synthesis can be measured over several days or even weeks, since the technique is not as sensitive to perturbations, such as food intake during the period when protein synthesis is measured. In recent years, the first studies have been published using this method in conjunction with resistance training, and the method is likely to become more common in the coming years [25].

Protein degradation

Resistance training leads to a positive protein balance, which allows for muscle hypertrophy. Although the positive protein balance can result from both increased protein synthesis and decreased protein breakdown, it is generally agreed that protein synthesis makes the strongest contribution to the overall protein balance during resistance training. This is primarily because the changes in protein synthesis following resistance training (plus food intake) are much greater than the changes in protein breakdown. Food intake reduces protein breakdown by about 50%, and this effect is due to the hormone insulin. Thus, insulin decreases protein degradation, but it should be emphasized that a relatively low protein intake is required for this effect [26].

It should also be recognized that protein breakdown is not necessarily negative for muscle mass. Continuous breakdown of damaged proteins is necessary to prevent tissues from gradually degrading. These damaged proteins are replaced by new proteins. Another reason is that amino acids are used for the synthesis of other important components of the body, such as neurotransmitters, hormones, and various peptides. Amino acids can also be used as energy substrates via acetyl–CoA or as intermediates in the Krebs cycle. In addition, the carbon skeleton of certain amino acids can be used for the synthesis of glucose (gluconeogenesis), ketone bodies (ketogenesis), or fat (lipogenesis).

Protein degradation is more difficult to measure compared to protein synthesis. There are both dynamic and static techniques for estimating protein degradation. The dynamic techniques rely mainly on tracers (stable isotopes). The static methods measure changes in molecular signals in muscle biopsies.

One difficulty with the dynamic measurements of protein degradation is that they assume that the efflux of the labeled amino acid into the venous blood represents the degradation. It is difficult to account for the degraded amino acids that remain in the muscle cells and are reused for protein synthesis. Therefore, the true extent of protein degradation may be underestimated. However, newer techniques have been developed to also account for amino acids in the intracellular pool.

Another marker of protein degradation is the myofibrillar protein degradation factor 3–methylhistidine (3MH). However, one problem is that 3MH can be derived from both cardiac and smooth muscle. Another drawback is that 3MH is usually measured in the interstitial fluid (the fluid in the space between cells), so it is unclear how well it represents the protein degradation of muscle.

MUSCLE PROTEIN METABOLISM DURING RESISTANCE TRAINING

Changes in muscle protein metabolism in response to resistance training sessions are relatively well studied. In the hours following exercise, protein balance changes as both protein synthesis and protein breakdown are affected. The increase in protein synthesis peaks in the first few hours after the session and then decreases. A typical curve can be seen in Figure 4.1. Protein synthesis is usually increased for at least 24 hours after a typical resistance training session. In the untrained state, i.e., if you have never done any resistance training or have had an extended break from training, protein synthesis is elevated even longer. This is one of the reasons why it becomes more difficult to gain muscle mass if you have been training regularly for a long time. The increase in protein synthesis after training is simply more short–lived [27] (Fig. 4.2). However, the strong protein synthesis response in the untrained state not only promotes muscle growth. It also promotes the repair of damaged muscle proteins caused by muscle damage [28].

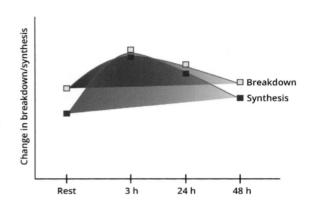

Figure 4.1.
Protein synthesis and protein breakdown in the fasting state at rest and up to 48 hours after resistance exercise. The figure shows that the increase in muscle protein synthesis is more pronounced and long–lasting than the increase in protein breakdown. However, the net balance in the fasted state is negative until amino acids (protein) are consumed in the diet. The figure is based on data from Phillips et al. 1997. The complete reference can be found in the Figure references section at the end of the book.

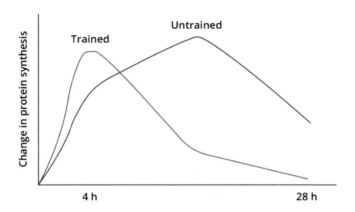

Figure 4.2.
Protein synthesis after resistance exercise in the untrained and trained state. The figure shows that the increase in muscle protein synthesis is more long–lasting in the untrained state. The figure is based on data from Tang et al. 2008. The complete reference can be found in the Figure references section at the end of the book.

Protein breakdown also increases after resistance training, yet for a shorter time compared to protein synthesis. It is estimated that protein breakdown peaks within a few hours after exercise and then returns to baseline levels within 24 hours [29]. Thus, as shown in Figure 4.1, the net protein balance in muscle, i.e., the difference between protein synthesis and protein breakdown, is negative in the fasting state. When amino acids are supplied through the diet, protein synthesis is greater than protein breakdown (Fig. 4.3). Nevertheless, it is wrong to claim that resistance training "breaks down" muscles because it is in fact the priming effect of resistance training that makes the protein balance positive compared to a normal day of rest. Resistance training should therefore be considered a fundamentally anabolic process.

Figure 4.3.
Muscle protein balance on two different days with or without resistance training. On a normal day, the rate of protein synthesis and protein breakdown are comparable (day 1). If you do resistance training and consume protein at some point during the day, protein synthesis exceeds protein breakdown (day 2). Thus, the net protein balance becomes positive due to the anabolic effect of resistance training.

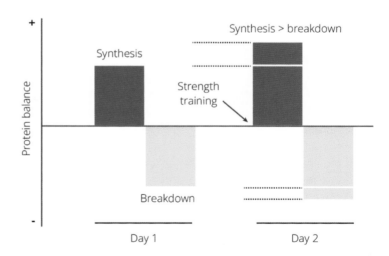

The molecular mechanisms controlling muscle protein turnover during and after resistance training are only partially known and involve many different signaling pathways. Alterations occur in gene expression, protein translation, as well as various molecular programs for protein degradation. The regulation of protein metabolism is discussed in more detail in Chapter 7.

The use of acute protein synthesis measurements, for example, to draw conclusions about the effects of various training programs or nutritional supplements has both advantages and disadvantages. One disadvantage is that the immediate increase in protein synthesis does not always correlate with the subsequent increase in muscle mass [30], especially at the beginning of a training program [31]. Furthermore, measurements are always limited by the biopsy time points chosen in the study. Protein synthesis and breakdown fluctuate up and down throughout the day, and the snapshots captured by the biopsies may simply not be representative of total muscle protein turnover.

Although a controlled training study can be considered "the truth" about whether an intervention influences muscle mass, there are drawbacks to these studies. Training studies are expensive and time–consuming to conduct, and it can sometimes be difficult to recruit subjects willing to donate repeated muscle biopsies. Training studies therefore often have low statistical power because of the small number of participants. This leads to difficulties in detecting small but potentially relevant differences between different interventions. In this case, an acute measurement with a larger number of subjects, e.g., in a cross–over design, has a greater potential to detect differences between interventions that can later be tested in a training study.

SUMMARY

- Protein turnover is an ongoing process that involves protein synthesis (in which amino acids are used to build new proteins) and protein breakdown (in which proteins are degraded to amino acids).

- Unlike fat and carbohydrates (glycogen), there are no protein stores that can be built up when protein intake is high. The small free circulating amino acid pool consists mainly of the newly digested amino acids.

- The protein turnover of skeletal muscle is estimated to be about 1–2% per day.

- The body's nitrogen balance provides only a general indication of whether the body is in an anabolic or catabolic state. It does not provide information on skeletal muscle protein turnover.

- Labeled amino acids – "amino acid tracers" – are often used to estimate muscle protein synthesis.

- A more recent technique for studying protein synthesis is the use of deuterium oxide, also called heavy water. The main difference between this technique and the use of amino acid tracers is that protein synthesis can be measured over several days or even weeks.

- There are both dynamic and static techniques for estimating protein degradation. There are several difficulties associated with measuring protein breakdown that limit these types of measurements in resistance training studies.

- The positive protein balance achieved by resistance training may be due to both increased protein synthesis and decreased protein breakdown, but protein synthesis is more important to the net protein balance than protein breakdown.

- Resistance training results in increased protein synthesis that lasts 24–72 hours.

- The increase in protein synthesis tends to be short–lived in the trained state.

- Protein breakdown is increased for a shorter time than protein synthesis after resistance training.

- Protein breakdown is an essential process, as proteins must be replaced to prevent gradual tissue deterioration.

- After resistance training, the net muscle protein balance is negative until dietary amino acids are supplied.

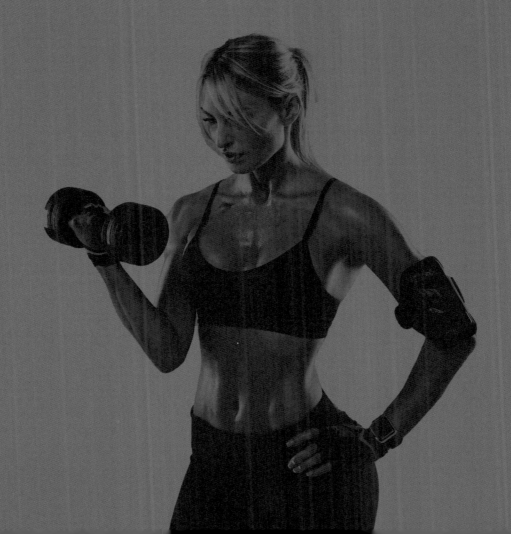

PART 2

ADAPTATIONS TO RESISTANCE TRAINING

05

CHAPTER 05

NEUROMUSCULAR ADAPTATIONS

Given that only a few training sessions can be sufficient to increase muscle strength, there must be other factors besides muscle hypertrophy that contribute to increasing strength. The answer lies in part in the interaction between the muscles and the nervous system, usually referred to as neural (or neuromuscular) adaptations. At the beginning of training, the neural adaptations include learning effects and more efficient execution of the specific exercises. Relatively quickly, however, muscle activation controlled by the nervous system improves, resulting in significant strength gains early in the training program. In this chapter, the most important neural adaptations in resistance training are presented.

STRENGTH GAINS

The most established adaptation to resistance training is the increase in muscle strength. Maximal strength (1RM) in a given exercise can be increased by three different mechanisms. First, a lifter can achieve greater efficiency by mastering the exercise and improving technique. This involves refining the interplay between agonists, synergists, and antagonists, which is called intermuscular coordination. This increase in strength occurs without a corresponding improvement in the intrinsic ability of the muscles to generate force.

The other way to increase strength is to increase the maximum neural activation of the muscle. This is made possible by specific neural adaptations achieved by resistance training. The final way to improve strength is through morphological adaptations in muscles, connective tissues, and tendons that increase strength development.

How much and at what rate muscle strength increases is more difficult to determine because individual differences are considerable. To give an example: In a study that examined strength gains after a 12–week biceps training program in over 500 individuals, the change in strength between individuals varied from –32% to +149% [32]. As discussed in other parts of the book, genetics plays an important role in the individual training response. The extent of strength improvement also depends on the test used to evaluate strength. The increase will be greater if strength is tested in the same exercise in which the training was performed (principle of specificity). More non–specific tests will show a smaller increase in strength.

Unfortunately, there are few long–term studies (>3 months) on resistance training that can provide information on the time course of strength improvement. One commonly cited study measured increases in strength, muscle cross–sectional area, and muscle activation of the thigh muscles after 2, 4, and 6 months of resistance training in seven healthy men in their 30s [33] (Fig. 5.1). The results showed that the strength improvement was greatest in the first two months and then decreased. However, strength gains were similar in months two through four and four through six. The total strength gain (isometric maximum) was 25% after 6 months. Overall, this shows that strength can increase steadily during the first few months of a strength training program.

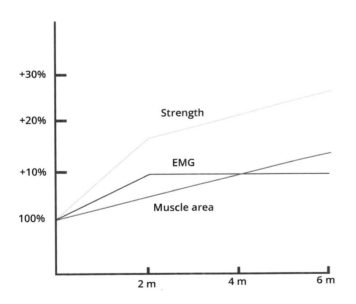

Figure 5.1.
Increase in muscle strength, neural activation measured by EMG, and muscle size measured by MRI during 6 months of resistance training. Based on data from Narici et al. 1996. The complete reference can be found in the Figure references section at the end of the book.

NEURAL ADAPTATIONS

Neural adaptations are greatest at the beginning of the training program when the rate of increase in strength is greatest. The role of the nervous system begins in the brain when the intended movement is planned. There, signals from different parts of the brain converge and together influence the final signal from the motor cortex to the spinal cord. The endpoint of the neural system is the neuromuscular junction, where the nerve end meets the muscle fiber.

When a person begins a resistance training program, whether as a beginner or after a long break from training, a large increase in maximum strength can be observed after only a few weeks. As indicated earlier, much of this increase in strength is due to neural factors. In the first weeks of training, strength usually increases in parallel with an increased EMG signal in the muscle. After a while, however, the neural adaptations diminish, and it becomes increasingly difficult to increase strength substantially.

The most important neural adaptation is the increased activation of the agonists (the muscles primarily activated during exercise). Another adaptation is the coordinated activation pattern of the synergists, while the antagonists resist the intended movement no more than necessary to protect the joint. The neuromuscular system also learns to process sensory feedback from the muscles and joints (proprioception). A summary of the most important neural adaptations can be found in Figure 5.2.

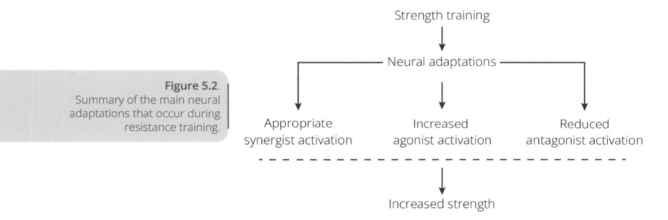

Figure 5.2. Summary of the main neural adaptations that occur during resistance training.

Evidence of neural adaptations

Most of the evidence for neural adaptations resulting from resistance training is quite indirect. The large strength gain compared to muscle growth at the beginning of a training program is often cited as evidence for neural adaptations. It is unrealistic that muscular factors, such as muscle hypertrophy, could contribute to a large increase in muscle strength in such a short time.

Another indirect evidence is the observation that the increase in strength is specific to the exercise performed (the principle of specificity). An example of this is that the increase in dynamic force is significantly greater than the increase in isometric force when the exercise is performed dynamically. Other indirect evidence of neural adaptations is that increases in strength are observed in the opposite, untrained arm or leg when the exercise is performed unilaterally (so-called cross-over or cross-education effect), or that imagined muscle contractions can produce a training effect.

The most concrete evidence of neural adaptation is the increased EMG signal that can be measured after several weeks of resistance training. An increase in the electrical signal in the muscle shows that the muscle is more activated by the nervous system.

The size principle

Henneman's size principle states that motor units are recruited in a specific order, from smallest to largest. The greater the voluntary effort, the more motor units are recruited to perform the desired muscle work. In practice, this means that the recruitment of motor units increases, either because the load (weight or resistance) increases or because the muscle is fatigued and needs to recruit even more motor units to maintain or increase strength. Since the small motor units innervate type 1 fibers, they are recruited first. This is followed by the type 2A and 2X fibers.

The question of whether the fast fibers can be recruited selectively, for example, during ballistic strength exercises, has been debated, but the general consensus is that the size principle also applies in these situations. Nevertheless, large motor units can be recruited with a lower force (lower recruitment threshold) in these types of actions [34].

AGONIST ACTIVATION

The most obvious neural adaptation following resistance training is increased activation of agonist muscles. Both the outer layer of the brain (cortical) and the areas beneath it (subcortical) undergo adaptations in response to resistance training to facilitate this. These adaptations work together to increase motor neuron activation, which in turn increases neural drive. This increased neural drive is a key mechanism behind the strength gains observed during training. These adaptations include changes in the plasticity of the motor cortex and spinal cord, as well as changes in the activation of motor units [35].

In the brain, changes in excitation and inhibition levels within motor circuits occur in the primary motor cortex. One way to measure the total motor output of the alpha motor neuron pool is the volitional or V-wave. An increase in V-wave amplitude following resistance training is often considered evidence of greater efferent drive and increased activation of the motor neuron pool.

A clear indication of the increased muscle activation is the increase in the firing rate of the motor units (**_rate coding_**). Through this mechanism, a motor unit can vary its force considerably, and increased rate coding with resistance training leads to increased force production (Fig. 5.3).

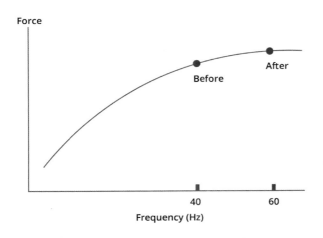

Figure 5.3.
Muscle force is increased from before to after training by increased firing frequency (rate coding). Increased rate coding is a prominent feature in adaptations to resistance training.

Another way to increase activation involves a combination of rapid recruitment of motor units and high firing frequency. If the intention is to contract the muscle as quickly and explosively as possible, such as during ballistic exercises, the motor units can be recruited more rapidly and also begin to fire action potentials at a very high frequency. The maximum firing rate achieved in this way is greater than that needed to achieve maximum force in a contraction. What happens is that the early rate of force development is increased, even if it is maintained for only a few milliseconds [36]. Thus, there is a training effect of achieving the highest possible recruitment and firing frequency of the motor units at the very beginning of a maximal contraction.

The maximal firing frequency can be 100–200 Hz during an explosive contraction, compared with 20–30 Hz during maximal force development during a contraction of steadily increasing intensity [37]. However, the rapid initial firing occurs only during a few pulses of action potentials. Firing frequencies of up to 50 Hz at maximal force development have been demonstrated during electrical stimulation, suggesting that the capacity to improve this ability through resistance training is relatively large.

Most of the evidence for increased agonist activation comes from EMG studies. The most studied muscle is the quadriceps femoris, which is the muscle group on the front of the thigh. From these studies, it appears that:

- ➲ EMG signal increases with resistance training
- ➲ Not all muscles respond in the same way
- ➲ Muscle activation depends on exercise intensity, volume, frequency, movement pattern (type of exercise), type of muscle action, and similarity between the test and the exercise performed (according to the principle of specificity)

The fact that neural adaptations are specific to the type of exercise performed was clearly demonstrated in a Finnish study from the mid–1980s [38,39]. After subjects completed a training program based on explosive jumps, maximum force increased by 11%, while the rate of force development increased by 24%. The increase in the rate of force development paralleled increased neural activation (rapid EMG increase). In contrast, during a strength program with traditional weights, maximum force increased by 27%, while the rate of force development remained unchanged. This indicated that the increase in the rate of force development during jump training was the result of specific neural adaptations resulting from explosive training.

Recruitment vs. rate coding

Which factor contributes most to increased agonist activation, increased recruitment, or increased rate coding? This depends in part on the type of action performed and the muscle group used [40]. For example, in small hand muscles, motor unit recruitment is rarely increased after 50–60% of maximum force. For most muscles, the upper limit of motor unit recruitment is ~85% of maximal force [41]. The increase of muscle force beyond the upper limit of motor unit recruitment is achieved by rate coding (Fig. 5.4). Under untrained conditions, therefore, there should be great training potential in increasing firing rate and thus increasing force rapidly. During the first few weeks of resistance training, however, increased agonist activation is usually mediated by adaptations in both motor unit recruitment and rate coding [42]. In particular, the physiological variation in the rate at which motor units are recruited during fast contractions is an important determinant of variability in how fast the force increases in different individuals [43].

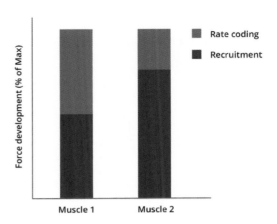

Figure 5.4.
Strategies for increased agonist activation. The relative contribution of recruitment versus firing frequency may differ between different muscle groups.

A CLOSER LOOK: Neural muscle activation

Activation of muscles by the nervous system can be measured by electromyography (EMG), in which electrodes are placed on the skin surface of muscles. Whereas early use of this surface electrode technique did not distinguish whether the electrical signal was from fiber recruitment or firing frequency, newer techniques have been developed to study the firing rate of individual motor units [44]. Although recording the activity of a single motor unit during a voluntary contraction is relatively straightforward today, assessing the effects of a long–term intervention is more difficult [41]. Apart from the technical challenge of identifying individual motor units, comparing their function before and after an intervention requires a sufficiently large sample and an adequate number of measurements. Therefore, few studies have examined the behavior of motor units before and after resistance training. In addition, the surface electrode technique is limited to studies of superficial muscles. More information can be obtained with intramuscular EMG electrodes because the electrodes are inserted into the muscle. However, these techniques have not been used to the same extent in resistance training studies. Given these limitations, it is difficult to directly use EMG information to evaluate the effectiveness of a particular exercise in promoting strength gains or muscle hypertrophy.

Another option for assessing muscle activation is functional magnetic resonance imaging (functional MRI). This technique examines the rapid fluid shifts that occur in active muscles during physical work. The more a muscle was used during a workout, the more fluid it absorbs because more metabolic products with osmotic properties were produced. The increased water content of the active muscles can be detected in the acquired MRI images.

With larger muscle groups, more and more motor units are recruited until maximum strength levels are approached. Even in the untrained state, about 90% of the available motor units can be recruited. Enhanced agonist activation for these muscle groups consists of a combination of increased recruitment and increased firing frequency. Concrete evidence for increased recruitment is difficult to provide because it would require demonstrating that a group of previously inactive motor units can be recruited following the training period.

The ability to maximally activate agonists may also vary between different muscle groups. For example, arm flexors have been shown to be more activated compared with quadriceps during maximal contraction

[45]. Most studies indicate that neural activation is rarely or never fully maximized. Nevertheless, the neural adaptations that lead to increased agonist activation are greatest at the beginning of an exercise program. After only 12 weeks, there may no longer be a significant improvement in agonist activation [46].

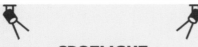

SPOTLIGHT
Can we activate all motor units?

· ·

Several studies that have investigated motor unit recruitment during resistance training show that we are unable to activate all available motor units despite maximal effort. This is studied using the interpolated twitch technique, in which a strong electrical stimulus is applied to the muscles during maximal contraction. Experiments using this method have shown that an additional force increase of about 5% is obtained immediately after stimulation [47], suggesting the recruitment of additional motor units. Nevertheless, both the maximal recruitment level and the recruitment rate may increase with training. In combination with an increased firing rate, these elements together enhance the activation of the agonist muscle.

Synchronization of motor units

It is controversial and has been questioned whether strength gains can be accompanied by an increase in synchronization of motor units., i.e., the timing of the firing of action potentials from active motor units. If there is a potential training effect in firing action potentials more synchronously, this could theoretically lead to increased force development. There are individual studies, both cross–sectional and longitudinal, that suggest that this synchronization of motor units occurs as a result of resistance training [48].

However, it is uncertain how important this synchronization of motor units actually is for the ability to produce maximal force, as studies have shown that synchronization does not contribute to further increases in force when the firing rate is already at the level of a maximal contraction [37]. It may be applicable to ballistic performance tasks, where the rate of force development is critical. Some studies have also shown that "duplets" of action potentials at intervals of less than 5 milliseconds are possible when large forces are to be generated rapidly [16].

NEUROMUSCULAR INHIBITION

Receptors in the muscles and tendons can give negative feedback to motor neurons in the spinal cord, reducing muscle activation by reducing central drive. This is considered a protective mechanism aimed at reducing excessive forces that can lead to injury. An example of this inhibition being effective is during maximal eccentric muscle actions. Theoretically, the muscle can generate more force during eccentric actions than during isometric or concentric actions. However, the maximum eccentric force generated is usually comparable to the maximum isometric force. Thus, it seems almost impossible to reach the theoretical upper limit of force during eccentric actions.

It has been found that this neural inhibition is less pronounced in trained powerlifters and can be somewhat reduced by electrical stimulation [49,50]. Heavy resistance training can also reduce this inhibition and thus increase force output [51]. This provides additional support for the hypothesis that neural inhibition is a protective mechanism in which inhibitory signals dampen the maximum possible activation.

Co-activation of antagonists

The role of the antagonists during a movement is to protect the joints from excessive forces and rotations. Contraction of the antagonists results in decreased force in the direction of movement while decreasing the ability to fully activate the agonists through reciprocal inhibition. Reciprocal inhibition means that activation of the agonists automatically decreases as the muscle on the opposite side of the joint contracts. Resistance training leads to better coordination between agonists and antagonists so that antagonist activation decreases, and strength development can increase. This effect is greatest at the beginning of a training program but can be continuously improved over long training periods [46].

RATE OF FORCE DEVELOPMENT

An important adaptation to resistance training is to increase the rate of force development. The rate of force development is the actual rate of force increase at the onset of a maximal muscle contraction; in other words, how fast the force increases. In most scenarios, this is almost synonymous with explosive force.

The rate of force development increases significantly after a period of explosive resistance training. For example, in one study, there was a 15% increase in the rate of force development after 14 weeks of resistance training [52]. This increase was associated with an increased EMG signal and an increased rate of EMG increase, which overall showed that neural drive had increased. Neural drive, which is the maximal ability to rapidly recruit and activate muscles, is an important factor in the rate of force development. In fact, the rate at which motor units are recruited appears to be the most important limiting factor for maximal rate of force development [43]. Other important factors are the composition of the fiber types, the ability to transmit force through the extracellular matrix, and the stiffness of the tendon.

Post Activation Potential (PAP)

A relatively recently discovered phenomenon is known as ***post-activation potentiation*** (PAP) [53]. PAP is a phenomenon in which the force exerted by a muscle during a contraction increases if it has been preceded by a previous contraction. Thus, the previous history of the contraction influences the execution of the subsequent muscle action. If these previous muscle contractions are performed with high loads over a few repetitions, this can lead to a subsequent increase in performance, especially in the form of an increased rate of force development. PAP can thus be considered a kind of preparatory warm-up in which the execution of a few explosive repetitions potentiates the subsequent acute performance. Various forms of plyometric jumps and heavy strength exercises seem to produce this phenomenon.

The proposed mechanisms that explain PAP mainly include three different theories. The first states that the preceding muscle contraction causes actin-myosin cross-bridges to be more sensitive to the release of calcium from the sarcoplasmic reticulum. The second theory is that there is increased synaptic excitation in the spinal cord, which leads to increased postsynaptic activation of the motor units that extend to the contracting muscles [54]. Finally, it has been suggested that a direct change in the pennation angle of the muscles may contribute to the phenomenon of PAP. Based on how PAP works, it can be concluded that the short-term potentiation of force development that can be achieved with this method primarily favors activities in which immediate force production is important, such as a sprint or a jump.

SUMMARY

- Regular resistance training leads to an increased ability to develop strength through neural and muscular adaptations.

- The increase in muscle strength is greatest in the beginning of a training program. How quickly, how much, and for how long strength can be increased depends on a number of different factors, including training status, training design, and genetic factors.

- There is both indirect and direct evidence of neural adaptations following resistance training.

- During resistance training, motor units are recruited in an order based on the size of motor neurons, from smallest to largest (the size principle).

- The most obvious neural adaptation after resistance training is increased activation of agonist muscles.

- Increased activation of agonists can be achieved by increased recruitment of motor units as well as increased firing frequency (rate coding) of individual motor units.

- Which of these factors contributes most to increased agonist activation depends in part on the exercise performed and the muscle group involved.

- It is controversial whether resistance training improve synchronization of motor unit firing patterns.

- While there is a phenomenon of neural inhibition that protects joints from high forces, heavy resistance training may reduce this neural inhibition to some degree, leading to increased force production.

- Resistance training leads to better coordination between agonists and antagonists so that antagonist activation decreases and force development can increase.

- The ability to produce force rapidly is referred to as the rate of force development, and neural adaptations mediate this increased rate of force development.

- Post–activation potentiation (PAP) is a phenomenon in which the force exerted by a muscle increases when a strong (but non–fatiguing) contraction has previously occurred.

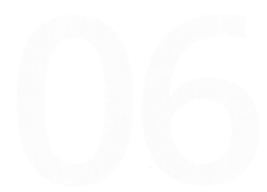

CHAPTER 06

HYPERTROPHY

Resistance training for many is synonymous with muscle growth – hypertrophy. The biological basis of muscle hypertrophy is probably more difficult to decipher than most people realize, largely because of limitations in study techniques. Muscle hypertrophy can be attributed to the enlargement of individual muscle fibers, an increased number of these fibers called hyperplasia, or even theoretically to the increased presence of connective tissue and other noncontractile material within or surrounding the muscle. Beyond these basic concepts, the process of muscle growth is multifaceted and influenced by numerous variables. This chapter addresses our current understanding of both the nuances and fundamentals of muscle hypertrophy.

MEASURING MUSCLE HYPERTROPHY

Muscle hypertrophy can be estimated using a variety of techniques, including simple measurements of muscle circumference with a tape measure or more precise diagnostic tools that measure cross–sectional area or volume, such as magnetic resonance imaging (MRI) and computed tomography (CT). At the fiber level, the cross–sectional area of individual fibers can be measured, and the amount of various muscle proteins quantified.

There are several assessment methods for estimating the anatomic cross–sectional area of muscle. Physiological cross–sectional area (a cross–section measured perpendicular to the fiber direction) may be an even better measure of the muscle's force capacity, but such measurements are complicated because they require determination of the muscle volume along with information on pennation angle and fiber length.

An important point is that measurements of cross–sectional area or muscle volume at the whole muscle level have much greater reproducibility than measurements at the fiber level. This is because fiber–level measurements are obtained from small muscle biopsies that may not be representative of the whole muscle.

Measurements that have been used to assess muscle hypertrophy in response to mechanical overload include [55,56]:

- **Mean/individual fiber cross–sectional area:** measured by histological staining and image analysis of muscle cross–sections. Increased fiber area indicates growth of muscle fibers.

- **Muscle thickness:** Measured by ultrasound at specific anatomical points (e.g., mid–thigh). May indicate hypertrophy of a muscle or muscle group.

- **Muscle volume:** Quantified by MRI or CT. Indicates the overall growth of a muscle.

- **Muscle cross–sectional area:** Measured by MRI or CT to assess the size of a muscle or muscle group at specific anatomical cross–sections.

- **Lean body mass:** Measured by dual–energy x–ray absorptiometry (DXA). Indicates the growth of lean mass (not fat/bone) of a body region.

Overall, a combination of microscopic and macroscopic techniques is likely required to fully characterize hypertrophy responses.

A CLOSER LOOK: Magnetic resonance imaging and computed tomography

. . . .

Images acquired with MRI are generally of the highest quality, and it is therefore possible to measure the area or volume of individual muscle bellies, e.g., all four individual quadriceps muscles. CT also provides relatively good image quality and is generally cheaper than MRI, but the examination is associated with a low radiation dose. Both MRI and CT measure the anatomic cross–sectional area (Fig. 6.1). Therefore, changes in architecture or physiological cross–sectional area of the muscle are not considered. However, an advantage of these imaging techniques is that the total muscle volume can be measured. The analysis usually requires manual measurement of the area image by image, which is very time–consuming. Recently, however, new techniques have been developed to automatically quantify the volumes of individual muscle groups based on a whole–body MRI scan [57]. It can be expected that this technique will have a great impact on body composition measurement in the future.

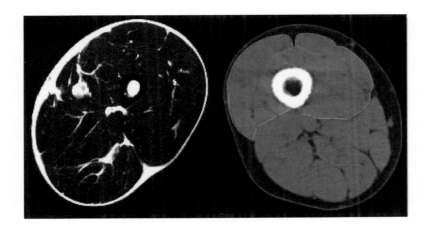

Figure 6.1.
Anatomical cross–sectional area of the thigh muscles with two different imaging techniques. The left image shows a magnetic resonance image (MRI), and the right image shows a computed tomography (CT) image. On the right image, the knee extensor (quadriceps) muscle group is circled.

TIME COURSE OF HYPERTROPHY

While muscle hypertrophy tends to be linear during the first few weeks or months of a resistance training program, it is obvious that at some point a plateau must occur. In one study, it was reported that bodybuilders did not increase muscle area or fiber size in response to 24 weeks of resistance training, providing some support for a plateau effect after many years of training [58]. Furthermore, in several studies in which muscle cross–sectional area was measured on more than one occasion, it was reported that muscle hypertrophy was greater in the first part of the training program than in the last part.

In the 6–month study mentioned in Chapter 5, muscle cross–sectional area increased relatively linearly throughout the training period [33]. In a study of elderly subjects, muscle thickness was examined after 6, 13, and 20 weeks of high or low–volume training. The results showed that higher training volume was important for muscle size to increase at the same rate by the end of the training period [59]. However, the increase was still linear in both training groups. Thus, it is still uncertain when the plateau effect will occur, and there are probably large differences between individuals. The design of the training program (volume, intensity, exercise selection, progressive overload) is likely to become increasingly important to ensure that muscle hypertrophy is sustained over a long period of time.

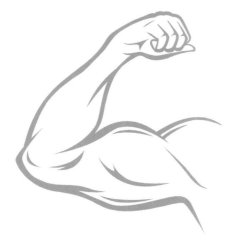

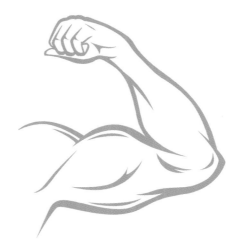

SPOTLIGHT
How fast can the muscle grow?

· ·

There are large individual differences in muscle mass gains from resistance training. Review articles and meta–analyzes report that muscle cross–sectional area increases by an average of 0.1–0.2% per day during shorter training periods [60]. However, these reviews included studies with large differences in important training variables such as exercise selection, volume, and intensity. Studies using optimized protocols and appropriate methods to measure muscle size have shown that the growth rate in the first few weeks of a resistance training program can be as high as 0.4% per day [61,62].

An interesting question is how much total muscle mass can be gained in a given period of time. It is difficult to give a clear answer to this question because several assumptions must be made. Uncertain factors include how much of the total muscle mass can be effectively trained and how much the degree of trainability differs between different muscle groups. We know with certainty that a "high responder" can increase thigh muscle mass by 20% in 5 weeks of training. The knee extensors in a 30–40–year–old male consist of about 2.5 kg of muscle mass. A 20% increase is equivalent to 500 grams of muscle mass. The total volume of muscle mass in the body is about 35 liters in a 180 cm tall man of the same age group. Assuming that muscle mass can increase by 1% per week in a high responder (averaged over all muscles), this results in an increase of just over 8 kg in 6 months. It is difficult to speculate on how realistic such a large increase in muscle mass is, but theoretically it should not be impossible.

HYPERPLASIA

The study of hyperplasia in humans, i.e., the process that leads to an increase in the number of fibers, is very difficult for methodological reasons. To establish hyperplasia beyond doubt, one would have to count the number of fibers in a muscle before and after a period of resistance training. This is, of course, impossible in humans, and it is also more or less impossible to make a good estimate from muscle biopsies taken before and after a period of training.

Some indirect attempts have been made to estimate hyperplasia by comparing fiber area between bodybuilders with many years of training experience and control subjects. Surprisingly, in a Swedish study from the 1980s, bodybuilders did not have significantly larger fibers than control subjects, and it was suggested that bodybuilders may have experienced hyperplasia as a result of years of training [63]. However, it could also be a selection bias in which individuals with many fibers are genetically predisposed to resistance training. This is similar to marathon runners, who have more slow fibers than sprinters. The main reason for this is probably genetic factors and the selection of a sport that fits one's genetic predisposition.

In the above study, it is also uncertain whether the fibers of the bodybuilders had actually divided or whether the fibers had simply not fully regenerated and were therefore misjudged in the microscope [64]. In other studies, the fiber area was significantly larger in bodybuilders than in untrained or moderately trained individuals [65], suggesting that hypertrophy of individual fibers is still the primary mechanism even with long–term training.

In animal models, it is possible to better estimate the number of fibers by comparing the number of fibers between an untrained and a trained limb. However, it must first be established that the number of fibers generally does not differ between the two limbs. There is at least one study that has done this [66]. The authors concluded that there was no difference in the number of fibers between the trained limb and the control group, which contradicts the hypothesis of hyperplasia.

In models in which birds were subjected to severe stretching, there is more concrete evidence of hyperplasia [67]. However, in the studies in which hypertrophy was produced by various methods of mechanical overload, the evidence is not as convincing. In the case of muscle growth from resistance training, there is no direct evidence of hyperplasia, although a recent review paper hypothesized that fiber splitting may be possible in extreme loading models [68].

A study conducted in Sweden in the early 1990s examining the number of fibers in the arm muscles of deceased subjects provided some evidence of limited hyperplasia in humans [69]. All seven subjects were right-handed and had larger right arms. Interestingly, the researchers were also able to count a significantly larger number of fibers in the right arm. These results suggest that prolonged, repetitive mechanical stress can lead to limited hyperplasia in humans. However, in the context of resistance training, the conclusion remains that hyperplasia is not a primary mechanism for muscle hypertrophy.

HYPERTROPHY OF INDIVIDUAL FIBERS

The increased cross-sectional area of individual muscle fibers is considered the main mechanism for whole-muscle hypertrophy during resistance training. The only way to properly assess fiber area is to take muscle biopsies. Usually, only a few hundred fibers can be assessed from a biopsy cross-section, which means that this method is associated with a large variance. Indeed, fiber hypertrophy can range from 10–50% in various studies that have assessed fiber hypertrophy in response to various interventions.

Type 2 fibers hypertrophy slightly more than type 1 fibers during resistance training, with fiber volume increasing primarily due to an increased number of contractile proteins. In a very time-consuming study, MacDougall and colleagues examined the density of myosin filaments in over 500 myofibrils from each subject. It was found that density was very constant both between individuals and when biopsies were compared before and after resistance training [70]. Thus, resistance training generally does not generally result in a more dilute protein fraction. Instead, the increased amount of contractile material causes the fibers to grow.

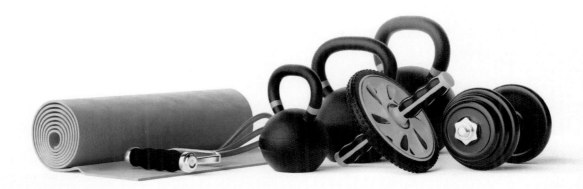

SPOTLIGHT
Does sarcoplasmic hypertrophy exist?
· ·

There are anecdotal observations that suggest bodybuilders have larger muscles than powerlifters, but are not as strong. To explain this, some older studies using electron microscopy suggested that resistance training leads to muscle growth by also increasing the sarcoplasmic space between myofibrils rather than increasing contractile proteins. This has been termed sarcoplasmic hypertrophy [71]. In support, Haun et al. reported that short–term high–volume resistance training can decrease actin and myosin protein concentrations in muscle fibers despite an increase in fiber size [72].

This notion of disproportionate sarcoplasmic expansion is still controversial, and several of the supportive studies have important limitations. Several lines of evidence argue against sarcoplasmic hypertrophy as the main mechanism, and it should be remembered that a large number of longitudinal studies have shown that specific tension is maintained in myofibers that have undergone growth as a result of increased mechanical loading [73]. This suggest that contractile proteins scale proportionally during muscle fiber growth [56,73]. However, there are still few ultrastructural data on subcellular adaptations during hypertrophy in humans. Very few studies have used electron microscopy to examine how organelles such as sarcoplasm, mitochondria, and myofibrils change during resistance training.

Overall, sarcoplasmic hypertrophy is a debatable concept, with most evidence supporting a proportional increase in contractile proteins and other intracellular components during muscle growth. However, this area needs further investigation using modern microscopic techniques.

A CLOSER LOOK: Fiber area
· · · · · · · · · · · · · · · · ·

Fiber area is usually measured under the microscope from cross–sections of muscle biopsies using histochemical techniques. If muscle hypertrophy results from more contractile elements being packed into the existing fibers, this will result in a parallel increase in fiber area. It should be noted, however, that this technique cannot account for whether the changes in fiber area depend precisely on the increase in contractile elements or whether there have been changes in noncontractile elements or increased packing of filaments within the same area. However, as discussed earlier, most of the available research suggests that the concentration of myofibrillar proteins is relatively constant in models that produce both severe hypertrophy and marked atrophy.

Although fiber area is a good measure of hypertrophy, there are several problems and limitations with this measurement. The most obvious is that it is impossible to measure all the fibers in the muscle. One must rely on a very small sample in the form of a muscle biopsy. To make matters worse, it is not possible to take biopsies from all the muscles in the body. These limitations reduce the reliability of fiber area measurements [74]. To obtain a reliable measure of muscle hypertrophy at the fiber level, the study should be performed on a large number of subjects, and preferably on many fibers and from multiple biopsies within the same subject. This is important to obtain a representative fiber distribution in the muscle studied, but also because there may be regional differences in the hypertrophy of a trained muscle. In reality, very few, if any, human research studies meet these criteria.

How are the new proteins packed into the muscle?

The contractile proteins myosin and actin make up the majority of proteins in the muscle cell, and these are the main proteins synthesized in the muscle after resistance training. But how are these new proteins packed into the fiber to become part of the contractile apparatus?

There is strong evidence that muscle size increases by both longitudinal and radial growth of fascicles. Most of the radial growth of muscle appears to be due to the enlargement of myofibrils, which increases the cross–sectional area of the fibers. However, it has not been conclusively determined whether this increase in size is due to the enlargement of individual myofibrils and/or the formation of new myofibrils.

In an extensive research review [73], the authors proposed a model called the "myofibril expansion cycle" to explain this process based on their analysis of existing research. According to this model, the cycle begins with the formation of new myofilaments around the outer portion of existing myofibrils, causing them to grow larger. When these myofibrils reach a certain size, they split into two smaller offspring myofibrils. These offspring myofibrils then enter the next round of the cycle, where they grow and divide again. This process continues and results in radial growth of the myofiber. Indeed, as new myofibrils are formed, consisting of new sarcomeres packed into the muscle either in parallel or in series, there is some evidence that the existing myofibrils grow in size. Studies with labeled proteins have shown that the new contractile proteins are mainly found in the periphery of the existing myofibrils [75].

As for the increase in the number of myofibrils, it is thought that the ruptures of the Z–discs caused by the obliquely pulling actin filaments allow the myofibrils to split. The newly synthesized contractile material is thus packed into the fibers in both existing and new myofibrils. The new sarcomeres are arranged both in parallel and in series, and since most muscles are pennate to varying degrees, adding both sarcomeres in parallel and in series results in an increase in muscle size. The architecture of the muscle is discussed in more detail in Chapter 9.

Fiber type changes

Most studies report no significant change in fiber type with resistance training. Significant in this context means that type 1 slow fibers are converted to type 2 fast fibers or vice versa. However, a general finding is that the proportion of type 2X fibers decreases in favor of type 2A fibers. This adaptation appears to occur in all types of exercise and thus is not specific to resistance training. Although this may seem odd given that the general goal of resistance training is to increase strength development, it must be remembered that the proportion of pure type 2X fibers in healthy, active people is extremely low to begin with. Moreover, neural adaptations, changes in muscle architecture, and preferential hypertrophy of type 2A fibers occur simultaneously to increase muscle strength. Interestingly, it appears that a period of detraining or unloading often results in a shift toward more 2X fibers [76]. Although further research is needed to clarify the significance of this phenomenon, it is a good example of the great plasticity of muscle tissue.

It is challenging to interpret the research on fiber types because there are many different techniques to classify fibers into different categories. For example, some researchers in the field claim that the pure fiber type 2X is found in only about 1% of all fibers [77]. Thus, many studies appear to report a misleadingly high percentage of type 2X fibers, likely due to differences in the various classification techniques used.

Another commonly reported finding is that the number of hybrid fibers, i.e., fibers expressing two or more different isoforms of the myosin heavy chain, decreases with resistance training. The relative proportion of hybrid fibers generally increases with age, also showing that fibers are plastic not only in response to exercise but also in response to decreased activity and during aging. Although there is no clear change in fiber type from the fastest to the slowest fibers and vice versa, fibers are still highly plastic as they metabolically and functionally adapt to the type of exercise being performed. Studies in mice have also shown that the same fiber can differ in composition along its longitudinal direction. This challenges our traditional view that a motor unit innervates only fibers of the same type.

DIFFERENCE BETWEEN MUSCLE GROUPS

Muscle hypertrophy is generally more pronounced in the muscles of the upper body than in the lower limbs in untrained individuals [78,79]. For example, in one study, the anatomical cross-sectional area of the biceps brachii in young subjects increased by 22% after 3 months of resistance training, whereas it increased by only 4–8% in the knee extensors and flexors [80]. The reason that the upper body muscles respond somewhat better to training may be related to the fact that many of the leg muscles have postural tasks, i.e., they help keep the body upright and are constantly activated in daily life. Therefore, they respond more poorly to resistance training compared to the arms. In addition, the arms generally have a higher proportion of type 2 fibers than the leg muscles [81].

EFFECT OF AGE

Older people do respond to resistance training and can increase their muscle mass. Even 90–year–olds have shown exceptional results, both in terms of increasing muscle mass and function [82]. When it comes to the question of whether the response to resistance training is attenuated in older individuals compared to younger individuals, the research is inconsistent and suffers from the fact that many studies are small and statistical power is low to detect minute differences. Overall, however, it appears that older people gain muscle mass at a slightly lower rate than younger people [83,84]. There are likely several reasons for this, which will be discussed in more detail in Chapter 17.

SELECTIVE HYPERTROPHY IN DIFFERENT MUSCLE GROUPS

The hypertrophy response may be different for different muscles within the same muscle group. The most studied muscle group is the knee extensors (quadriceps femoris). In this muscle group, the rectus femoris increases the most (in relative numbers), followed by the vastus lateralis, vastus medialis, and vastus intermedius (Fig. 6.2). The reason for the differences in hypertrophy between muscles is probably related to the activation pattern of the specific muscles during resistance training and to the composition and architecture of the muscle fibers.

The hypertrophic response may also vary with the anatomical direction of the muscle. In one study, the relative hypertrophy of the rectus femoris muscle differed by 10–50% depending on where the muscle size was measured [33]. In general, the quadriceps muscle seems to grow slightly more in the middle and distal parts than in the proximal part. This may explain why the increase in muscle size based on a single cross–sectional image does not correlate perfectly with measurements of the volume of the whole muscle [85]. This variation within and between muscles is one of the reasons why measurement of muscle volume is preferable when possible.

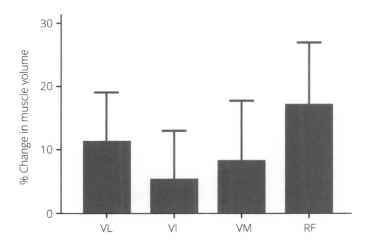

Figure 6.2.
The increase in muscle volume of the four individual quadriceps muscles after 5 weeks of resistance training. VL = vastus lateralis, VI = vastus intermedius, VM = vastus medialis, RF = rectus femoris. Based on data from Lundberg et al. 2019. The complete reference can be found in the Figure references section at the end of the book.

INDIVIDUAL VARIATION IN HYPERTROPHY

There are individual differences in how well we respond to resistance training in terms of increasing muscle mass and strength. Two seemingly comparable individuals may not achieve the same result even if they follow the same program. This is because there are several different factors that determine an individual's response to resistance training. Examples of factors that may be important include age, sex, training status, and genetics.

A clear example of the variation in muscle hypertrophy in response to training is shown in Figure 6.3. The subjects (10 young men) performed resistance training with the identical training program for the knee extensors (5 weeks, 12 sessions of 4 × 7 repetitions on a flywheel ergometer). As can be seen in the figure, there were large differences between participants in terms of muscle volume gains. Although it is generally accepted that some individuals respond very well to resistance training and others respond poorly, it is important not to draw too strong conclusions from individual studies. To properly study so–called "responders" and "low responders" to resistance training, experiments should be repeated with the same individuals to show that the results are reproducible and not just random variability or regression to the mean. Unfortunately, very few such studies have been conducted.

Figure 6.3.
Individual variation in muscle hypertrophy following an identical resistance training program (5 weeks for knee extensors). Each bar corresponds to one participant in the study. Based on data from Lundberg et al. 2013. The complete reference can be found in the Figure references section at the end of the book.

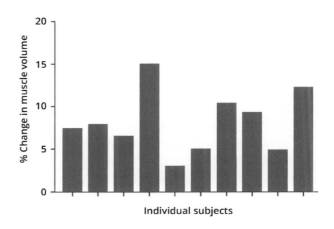

In a study of elderly subjects, it was reported that there were no non responders when a series of measures of muscle hypertrophy, strength, and physical function were considered [86]. Each participant improved at least one variable. This suggests that anyone can achieve a positive adaptation to resistance training, but some will have to work harder to do so. Although there may be no true "non responders," it is probably fair to say that there are low responders and high responders.

Of the various factors that may be important to an individual's response to resistance training, genetics appears to play the largest role. In the research literature examining high responders and low responders, findings include the following[87]:

- High responders have more satellite cells than low responders before training begins.
- Responders have a better ability to activate satellite cells and produce new myonuclei with resistance training.
- There may be differences between responders and low responders with respect to various gene polymorphisms, such as the ACTN3 gene.
- Differences in mitochondrial volume and capillary density have been found between responders and low responders.
- High responders have a better ability to increase the production of ribosomes in muscle cells (ribosome biogenesis).
- The magnitude of the increase in protein synthesis after an acute exercise session is greater in responders than in low responders.
- There may be differences in the expression of microRNAs between responders and low responders (microRNAs are discussed in Chapter 7).
- The basal gene expression profile, based on all genes expressed in muscle, may differ between responders and low responders.
- The amount of androgen receptors correlates with muscle hypertrophy and may differ between responders and low responders.

It should be noted that the above list contains several preliminary results that should be treated as hypotheses rather than established facts. Although the mechanisms explaining the interindividual response to resistance training appear to be largely related to genetics, we have so far had limited knowledge of the exact mechanisms. There are currently no reliable tests that can be used to determine an individual's resistance training potential. One of the simplest explanations for trainability is probably the composition of fiber types, with individuals having a high proportion of fast fibers responding better to resistance training than individuals having a high proportion of slow fibers.

In a study examining response to concurrent training, increases in single-leg cycling performance (incremental test to fatigue) and increases in muscle size after 5 weeks of both strength and endurance training were compared. There was a negative correlation between the increase in endurance performance and the increase in muscle size, suggesting that those who respond to endurance training generally respond worse to resistance training and vice versa (Fig. 6.4). In fact, the correlation in trainability "between" exercise modalities appears to be low[88], suggesting that most people can benefit from some type of exercise training.

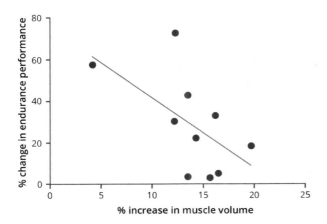

Figure 6.4.
The relationship between performance in an endurance test (single–leg cycling to exhaustion) and muscle volume increase during 5 weeks of combined strength and endurance training. Based on data from Lundberg et al. 2013. The complete reference can be found in the Figure references section at the end of the book.

DOES MUSCLE HYPERTROPHY CAUSALLY DETERMINE STRENGTH DEVELOPMENT?

Although there is a relatively strong correlation between baseline muscle size and strength, this does not necessarily mean that increases in muscle mass will cause increases in strength during a training program. This fact has been increasingly highlighted by various researchers in recent years [89]. It has been found that the correlation between the relative change in muscle mass and the change in strength after a training period is not as strong as one might think. The reason for this is probably that other factors affecting force production, not least neural adaptations, dominate during this period. However, this does not change the fact that a larger muscle is stronger than a smaller muscle when all other factors are equal. Increases in muscle mass during resistance training should, therefore, eventually translate into increases in strength.

SUMMARY

- ➲ An increase in muscle size, hypertrophy, results primarily from an increase in the size of individual muscle fibers.

- ➲ It cannot be ruled out that some hyperplasia occurs during resistance training, but the primary mechanism for muscle hypertrophy is the growth of individual fibers driven by an increased quantity of contractile material in the cells.

- ➲ Muscle hypertrophy begins immediately during resistance training, but it is unclear how long hypertrophy can continue at the same rate until a plateau occurs.

- ➲ How fast the muscle grows in response to resistance training varies greatly from person to person and can also vary between different muscle groups.

- ➲ Type 2 fibers hypertrophy more than type 1 fibers after resistance training.

- ➲ Existing myofibrils grow in size and number, while new contractile filaments and sarcomeres are packed into the muscle either parallel to each other or in series.

- ➲ Resistance training generally results in a reduction in the number of type 2X fibers in favor of type 2A fibers, while the proportion of hybrid fibers decreases.

- The composition of fiber types is strongly influenced by genetics.

- The large muscle groups of the arms grow slightly more than the muscle groups of the legs during resistance training.

- Even old people respond to resistance training with an increase in muscle mass and strength.

- The hypertrophic response of muscles may differ between different muscles within the same muscle group and may also vary in the anatomical direction of the muscle (regional differences).

- The ability to build muscle mass varies greatly between individuals, and there are a number of different proposed cellular and genetic mechanisms to explain why some people respond as "high responders" and others as "low responders" to resistance training.

- A larger muscle is stronger than a smaller muscle, but increases in muscle mass do not always correlate with increases in strength during short–term training periods.

07

MECHANISMS FOR HYPERTROPHY

The intricacies of muscle hypertrophy as it relates to resistance training are fascinating and complex. What causes muscle fibers to expand, and how do muscle fibers respond and adapt to mechanical loading? These processes are undoubtedly multifactorial, and our understanding of the mechanisms remains an evolving area of research. This chapter aims to explore these complex processes by explaining the main mechanisms currently thought to trigger and regulate hypertrophy.

STIMULI FOR MUSCLE HYPERTROPHY

The stimuli that trigger muscle hypertrophy in response to resistance training must come from processes set in motion by the mechanical loading on the muscle. It is difficult to pinpoint the most important factor because many signaling pathways interact and some are redundant. Stimuli and events thought to be important in triggering the anabolic response that leads to muscle hypertrophy include:

- Signals triggered by mechanosensors on the cell membrane or in proteins of the cytoskeleton (mechanical stress)
- Stretch of muscle fibers
- Metabolic stress
- Calcium signaling
- Free radicals
- Processes stimulated by hormones and other growth factors
- Muscle damage
- Cell swelling
- Activation of satellite cells

Mechanotransduction

Skeletal muscles have sensors that detect and transmit mechanical tension and translate this information into an anabolic response that favors protein synthesis. This cascade of cell signals is called mechanosensation or mechanotransduction. It is unlikely that a single factor is responsible for sensing and converting mechanical stress into an anabolic response. Several different mechanosensors are activated to varying degrees depending on the predominant stimulus acting on the muscle. However, our knowledge of these processes is quite limited. A recent review article highlighted filamin C–BAG–3–mediated regulation of mTOR as one of the key factors [90]. These proteins are associated with the Z–discs of muscle fibers. Other candidates include Costamere–related proteins, focal adhesion kinase, and phosphatidic acid.

Stretch of muscle fibers

It has long been known from animal models that fibers subjected to stretching are stimulated to grow. Since stretching of muscle fibers does not result in a major inflammatory cascade in the cells, the stretching method can be used to study early hypertrophy processes. It has also been reported that the stretching model leads to hyperplasia in animal models. In human hypertrophy studies, it is unclear whether stretching the fibers per se stimulates significant muscle growth [91], but, as in resistance training, stretching results in mechanical tension on extracellular components that activate mechanosensors in muscle fibers. Nevertheless, it appears that stretching muscle fibers in humans is significantly less effective than resistance training in eliciting a stimulus for muscle hypertrophy.

Metabolic stress

Bodybuilders often train with moderate loads and multiple sets and repetitions until muscular exhaustion (failure). The metabolic stress that occurs during such a program is considered a stimulus for muscle hypertrophy, but with limited evidence. Metabolic stress includes increased calcium turnover, accumulation of lactate and other metabolites, ischemia and hypoxia, and increased production of reactive oxygen species (free radicals).

Metabolic stress also occurs during endurance training. This is an example of the overlap between strength and endurance training. For example, increases in the metabolically responsive protein kinase AMPK have been associated with important adaptations in both strength and endurance training [92]. Nevertheless, the endpoint of adaptation in muscle typically differs between strength and endurance training. Overall, metabolic stress should be considered as a complement to perhaps the most important stimulus, mechanical tension, in the initiation of muscle hypertrophy.

Calcium turnover

Repeated muscle contractions are associated with a large load on calcium metabolism. During muscle contractions, calcium is constantly pumped into and out of the sarcoplasmic reticulum. There are several calcium–dependent signaling pathways in muscle cells, and calcineurin–mediated signaling has been shown to be associated with fiber hypertrophy. The calcineurin signaling pathway may interact with multiple signaling cascades that influence the initiation of muscle protein synthesis. Further evidence for its role is that inhibition of this pathway can prevent muscle growth, at least in mice [93].

Free radicals

The production of oxygen and nitrogen radicals, known as reactive oxygen species (ROS), increases with exercise. ROS have unpaired electrons in their outer shell and were previously considered harmful because they can negatively affect cell DNA. Today, we know that ROS can affect several important cellular signaling pathways involved in muscle adaptation to exercise. This is indirectly supported by studies showing that excessive intake of antioxidants, which dampen the production of ROS, can negatively affect muscle adaptations to training (see Chapter 14).

During resistance training, the production of ROS increases, which can stimulate local growth factors and affect gene expression 94. ROS can also stimulate increased production of cytokines, such as various interleukins. These cytokines play an important role in regulating muscle adaptation to exercise. However, there are no experimental studies demonstrating that free radical production is an absolute requirement for muscle hypertrophy.

Cell swelling

During resistance training, the production of metabolites in muscle fibers increases, attracting fluid through the process of osmosis. This means that water from the bloodstream enters the muscle and causes temporary swelling. The osmotic swelling effect could be a stimulus for muscle hypertrophy. This is supported by research showing that cellular swelling itself can trigger increased protein synthesis and decreased protein degradation [95]. It is thought that swelling leads to tension and pressure on the cell membrane, thereby initiating intracellular signaling cascades that promote anabolic processes. It has also been suggested that cell swelling leads to more efficient activation of satellite cells [96].

Exercise–induced muscle damage

It is often argued that exercise–induced muscle damage is a stimulus for muscle hypertrophy. However, increased muscle protein synthesis can be observed even in the absence of muscle damage, and muscle hypertrophy is also observed after resistance training programs that do not induce muscle damage. In a relatively recent training study, it was shown that muscle protein synthesis did not correlate with hypertrophy at the beginning of the program when muscle damage was pronounced. Instead, it took three weeks for protein synthesis to reflect the hypertrophic response [28]. It was concluded that the increase in protein synthesis at the beginning of a training program does not primarily drive muscle hypertrophy but rather contributes to the necessary remodeling of muscle fibers. After a few weeks of training, a correlation is observed between the increase in protein synthesis and the degree of hypertrophy. During this phase, muscle damage is usually very low. This indicates that muscle damage should not be considered the primary stimulus for muscle hypertrophy.

Hormones and other growth factors

Several circulating hormones can activate various anabolic processes and play a role in regulating muscle hypertrophy. By affecting target cell receptors, hormones can influence muscle protein synthesis and activate muscle stem cells (the satellite cells).

Testosterone, the male sex hormone, is often associated with muscle growth and many seem to believe that the release of testosterone is one of the most important mechanisms for muscle hypertrophy. However, this is not the case, although it is possible to stimulate muscle growth with high doses of testosterone [97]. This effect has been associated with increased activation of satellite cells and increased numbers of myonuclei [98].

However, even with reduced testosterone levels, muscle growth is still possible. For example, unchanged hypertrophy was observed in male castrated rats even though circulating testosterone levels decreased by 90% [99]. In humans, healthy men undergoing testosterone suppression show a hypertrophic response to resistance training [100], and it is known that women respond as well to resistance training as men despite very different testosterone levels [101].

More concrete evidence that circulating testosterone levels are not critical for muscle hypertrophy comes from experiments in which testosterone levels were increased first by sprint cycling and then by resistance training for the arms. This approach does not have a positive effect on the hypertrophy response, even though testosterone levels are much higher with this training setup than with resistance training alone [102].

There are other hormones that are thought to be important for muscle hypertrophy, including growth hormone (GH). GH acts by stimulating the insulin growth factor (IGF) system. However, in animal models, it is possible to completely block the receptor for IGF–1 and still observe intact muscle hypertrophy in response to mechanical overload [103].

Activation of satellite cells

The immature stem cells of the muscle, the satellite cells, are activated during a single resistance training session, and an increase in the number of satellite cells can be detected as early as 24–72 hours after [104]. The satellite cells are important for the regeneration of muscle fibers after injury and probably also after resistance training. However, the direct importance of satellite cells for muscle hypertrophy is controversial. This will be discussed later in this chapter.

THE ACUTE CELLULAR RESPONSE
TO RESISTANCE TRAINING

Acute resistance training results in an increase in muscle protein synthesis that lasts for 24–72 hours, depending on effort and training status. The increase in protein synthesis is mainly due to an increase in the rate of translation, where the mRNA code is translated into proteins. In addition, resistance training leads to changes in the expression of hundreds to thousands of genes. Many of these mRNAs have been shown to be "myogenic," meaning that they are involved in the muscle remodeling process. How this is coordinated and regulated is very complex, and it is difficult to link the response to a single training session to the long-term adaptive response.

It would be very attractive to find a gene or molecular signaling factor that could serve as a marker for the degree of muscle hypertrophy to be expected after resistance training. If this were possible, it would be relatively easy to compare different programs and interventions and determine, for example, the optimal combination of training and diet for different populations. Unfortunately, research to date has fallen far short of being able to assess the effectiveness of individual resistance training exercises based on these acute markers. Here are some examples that illustrate the problem of linking acute responses to the degree of muscle hypertrophy after training:

- The increase in muscle protein synthesis in the untrained state is considerably more long-lived than the increase in the trained state.

- The increase in protein synthesis is not necessarily linearly related to the increase in muscle mass after a period of resistance training.

- The increase in translational signaling is not linearly correlated with the increase in muscle mass after a period of resistance training, and in some cases, there is a marked divergence between signaling and protein synthesis.

- In the untrained state, endurance training and resistance training results in a similar molecular signaling response, even though resistance training results in more pronounced hypertrophy than does endurance training.

- Key factors for muscle hypertrophy in animal models have not been reproduced in human experiments.

As can be seen from the above, it is challenging to link the acute cellular response to the end product, i.e., muscle hypertrophy. To better understand the mechanisms that regulate muscle hypertrophy during resistance training, it is important for future research to clarify how the acute response is related to the degree of muscle hypertrophy during resistance training.

MOLECULAR REGULATION OF PROTEIN TURNOVER

In the chapter on muscle protein metabolism, it was described how muscle protein synthesis and breakdown vary throughout the day and how resistance training affects this balance. How are these processes, which ultimately control muscle hypertrophy, regulated?

The molecular response to resistance training is complex and involves events throughout the DNA code, from how our genes are turned on and off (mRNA expression) to how this code is translated into a functional protein in the ribosomes of the cell. Each individual training session leads to the activation of several different signaling cascades and simultaneously activates hundreds to thousands of genes (Fig. 7.1). Over time, these changes contribute to the accumulation of various muscle proteins.

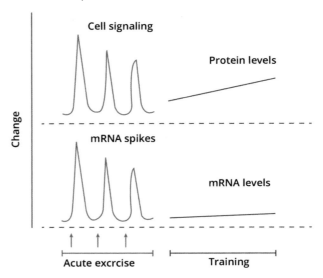

Figure 7.1.
Overview of changes in mRNA and protein levels in response to acute exercise and chronic training. Together, these molecular adaptations contribute to long-term performance improvement. The image has been redrawn following Egan & Zierath (2013). The complete reference can be found in the Figure references section at the end of the book.

DNA modifications and epigenetics

The regulation of gene expression is very complex and is not only determined by the genetic blueprint itself (i.e., DNA). For example, it has been found that non-genetic structural changes in DNA can affect gene expression. This can be considered an additional "layer" involved in regulating gene activity. The delivery of methyl groups to one or more nucleotides in the DNA molecule helps control how genes are turned on and off in response to various stimuli. This is known as epigenetics, and the associated DNA methylation has been shown to be affected by exercise [105]. However, exactly how epigenetic changes affect muscle hypertrophy remains to be elucidated.

Transcriptional regulation

The importance of transcriptional regulation of muscle hypertrophy was first demonstrated in experiments with the transcriptional inhibitor actinomycin D, which completely prevented plantar muscle growth in rats [106]. The transcriptional response is complex and difficult to link to muscle hypertrophy because the initial changes in mRNA expression are distinctly different from the longer-term changes that occur with repeated exercise (i.e., training).

Transcriptional regulation involves the binding of various transcription factors to the DNA strand, triggering the transcription of various target genes. Resistance training alters the expression of genes involved in a variety of functions, including cell growth, differentiation, inflammation, and protein degradation (proteolysis). Although the translation of mRNA to protein is thought to be the main regulator of increased protein synthesis after exercise, the gene expression response also affects protein turnover. Specific transcription factors are of particular importance in controlling the activity of different groups of genes (gene clusters).

A single bout of resistance training alters the transcription of several hundred genes in both trained and untrained states [107]. Using techniques such as microarrays or RNA sequencing, it is possible to examine how the whole genome, i.e., the expression of all genes in muscle, responds to exercise or how the transcriptome differs between different populations in cross-sectional comparisons. For example, differences in baseline expression of various genes have been found between individuals who respond well to resistance training and those who respond poorly (high and low responders).

One known factor that exerts its effect at the transcriptional level is myostatin. Increased expression of myostatin decreases muscle size, and myostatin is therefore a negative regulator of muscle hypertrophy. This has become known to the public through pictures of massive and muscular animals lacking the gene for myostatin, such as the "Belgian Blue" cattle. In humans, a case of a defective myostatin gene was discovered in a German boy in 2004, leading to extreme muscle size and strength [108]. During resistance training, a single exercise session leads to decreased expression of myostatin, promoting muscle hypertrophy.

Another example is the ubiquitin ligase proteins atrogin–1 and MuRF–1, which are thought to be regulated at the mRNA level. These proteins mark contractile proteins to be degraded. They are therefore closely associated with muscle atrophy in various unloading and atrophy models. However, studies have shown that increases in MuRF and atrogin–1 also occur in situations where muscle growth is occurring. This has led to the interpretation that they are involved in the normal post–exercise remodeling process in which some proteins must be broken down and replaced [109,110].

Recently, microRNAs (miRNAs) have been recognized as potentially important mediators of muscle adaptations to resistance training. miRNAs are noncoding sequences of mRNA that degrade various transcripts by binding to complementary sequences. Several miRNAs have the potential to affect different mRNAs [111], and several miRNAs have been shown to increase in response to exercise. It is therefore possible that these may influence the hypertrophic process [112].

A CLOSER LOOK: Gene Expression

Studying the activity of a gene or mRNA expression provides important information about how the gene functions and how its protein is regulated. Using various chemicals, RNA can be extracted from muscle tissue. After RNA extraction, there are several methods to study the mRNA. Quantitative real–time PCR (polymerase chain reaction) has been the most common method for studying specific mRNAs. This method is very sensitive and relatively fast. Specific primers are used to amplify the correct gene and determine the amount of product. It is more common today to measure the expression of all genes simultaneously using so–called arrays or RNA sequencing. Both methods provide information about the transcription of the entire genome. Increasingly, the research literature on resistance training analyzes the response of the entire genome rather than individual preselected genes.

Translational control

An increased rate of translation of mRNA into protein is an important explanation for why protein synthesis increases with resistance training. This was shown in early experiments with electrical stimulation of rat muscle [113]. After 48 hours, it was shown that the increase in protein synthesis was mainly due to increased translation of mRNA rather than increased mRNA quantity. Translation is an energy–consuming and tightly regulated process. Not all muscle proteins increase with resistance training. The contractile proteins are preferred, especially when the muscle has become accustomed to training.

The translation of mRNA into protein involves three distinct steps: Initiation, elongation, and termination. Of particular importance is the initiation step, which is coordinated by a protein complex called mTOR (mechanistic target of rapamycin). mTOR integrates signals originating from mechanical stimuli, energy status, and nutrients (mainly amino acids), and coordinates the various signaling pathways that lead to altered protein synthesis. Activation of mTOR promotes increased protein synthesis after resistance training and is considered a key factor in stimulating muscle hypertrophy [114].

Proteins downstream of mTOR include p70S6 kinase (p70S6K) and eukaryotic initiation factor 4E–BP1. In support of the role of these proteins in regulating protein synthesis, p70S6K was reported to correlate with an increase in muscle mass in electrically stimulated rats [115] and, additionally, after 14 weeks of resistance training in humans [116]. Increased mTOR signaling is often associated with increased protein synthesis after resistance training, as well as with an increase in muscle mass after prolonged training [117]. Therefore, translational control of protein synthesis is considered a critical step for muscle hypertrophy.

A CLOSER LOOK: Protein methods

In resistance training research, the amount of a particular protein in a muscle sample is often determined. The Western blot, or immunoblot, is the most common molecular biology technique for quantifying proteins. The proteins are first extracted from the muscle tissue. They are then separated on a gel based on their molecular mass, which affects how fast the proteins "run" in the gel. Specific antibodies can be used to label the protein of interest and quantify its amount (Fig. 7.2). Another common method based on the same principles is ELISA (Enzyme–Linked ImmunoSorbent Assay). The ELISA method has a greater capacity to analyze many samples and proteins, but with Western blot, one usually has greater control over what is measured because one can visually see the size of the protein, which reduces the risk of false–positive results. However, there are other sources of error and problems with Western blot that can be avoided with ELISA. Techniques have also been developed in the last decade to quantify most muscle proteins simultaneously. This research is still in its infancy but will likely provide important information about muscle adaptations to resistance training in the future.

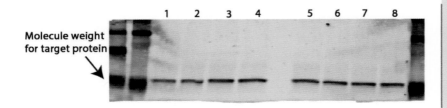

Molecule weight for target protein

Figure 7.2.
Western blot. Protein homogenates are added to the wells on the gel (1–8 in the figure) and separated according to their molecular weight. The size of each band represents the amount of protein in the sample and is detected with specific antibodies.

Ribosome biogenesis

Mechanical overload leads to an increase in ribosomal RNA and total RNA content in skeletal muscle. This reflects an expansion of ribosomes and translational capacity through the process of ribosome biogenesis. Increased formation and improved function of ribosomes are required for protein synthesis to continue to increase as muscle grows. Ribosomes are the organelles in which amino acids are linked together to form the newly built protein based on the mRNA blueprint. The rate-limiting step in ribosome biogenesis is thought to be the transcription of rDNA genes by RNA polymerase I and the subsequent formation of 45S pre–rRNA, the amount of which increases in response to hypertrophic stimuli [118].

Time–course data suggest that ribosome biogenesis occurs early in response to mechanical overload before measurable muscle hypertrophy is detected. Furthermore, the extent of ribosome biogenesis correlates with the degree of muscle growth induced by mechanical overload. This indicates that increased ribosome production precedes and enables the increased protein synthesis that underlies muscle fiber growth. By expanding translational capacity early in the process, ribosome biogenesis enables muscle cells to support the higher rates of protein synthesis required for hypertrophy. Thus, increased ribosome biogenesis is an important preparatory mechanism that enables skeletal muscle to undergo large–scale hypertrophy in response to the sustained protein synthesis demands of resistance training [56].

SATELLITE CELL ACTIVATION AND MYONUCLEI ACCRETION

Adding more myonuclei to fibers may be important for muscle hypertrophy because it helps maintain the ratio between the number of nuclei and cell volume. This is commonly referred to as the myonuclear domain theory. The theory is based on the notion that the ratio between fiber volume and the number of nuclei should be relatively constant so that the cell does not lose its ability to transcribe and synthesize proteins (Fig. 7.3).

Figure 7.3.
The myonuclear domain theory. According to this theory, the number of nuclei in muscle fibers should increase as the fibers increase in size during resistance training. The theory states that each nucleus is responsible for a certain volume of the fiber.

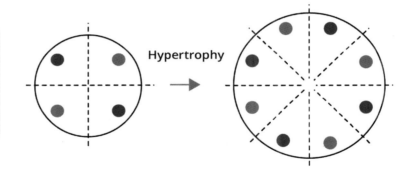

The process of myonuclei accretion is thought to be controlled primarily by the satellite cells located between the basal lamina and the sarcolemma. As mentioned earlier, the satellite cells are activated by resistance training and increase in quantity. It is believed that some of these satellite cells fuse with the muscle fiber during long–term training, becoming fully mature myonuclei. Since muscle cells do not undergo cell division, this is a mechanism that may explain the proliferation of myonuclei in muscle fibers.

The significance of satellite cell activation and subsequent myonuclear addition is controversial. Much of the early research was conducted in mice, and interpretations of these studies are compromised by the fact that the age of the mice appears to have a critical influence on the response [119]. In young, adolescent mice, the increase in muscle mass correlates with satellite cell activation and increased myonuclei content, whereas older mice show marked hypertrophy even though satellite cells are knocked out [120].

The role of satellite cells in the hypertrophy process in humans is supported by studies reporting that the number of nuclei is greater in strength–trained subjects compared with untrained controls. Moreover, in some studies, resistance training–induced fiber hypertrophy has been associated with increased numbers of satellite cells and myonuclei [121]. However, far from all resistance training studies have found an increase in the number of nuclei. Some researchers have hypothesized that an increase in myonuclei occurs primarily when a certain "upper limit" of muscle growth is reached. This upper limit would be at a fiber hypertrophy equivalent to about 20%.

However, a meta-analysis concluded that there is no clear evidence for a specific "hypertrophy ceiling" at which myonuclei growth is required. Nevertheless, it was found that an increased number of nuclei per fiber was more frequently observed in studies in which fiber hypertrophy was substantial [122].

In summary, resistance training can lead to the formation of more nuclei in muscle fibers, which is called myonuclear accretion. This may be important in supporting muscle hypertrophy by increasing the capacity for gene transcription. The type of training, the duration of the training period, and the methodology used to analyze myonuclear density may explain the partially conflicting data reported to date.

When we talk about myonuclei, the question of "muscle memory" usually comes up. This refers to the question of whether the muscle has a "memory" for previous training. It has been hypothesized that muscle fibers have imprints from previous training, which allows for faster rebuilding of muscle mass and strength. As early as 1991, the concept of muscle memory was discussed in a study in which both fiber area and muscle strength increased relatively rapidly during a 6-week retraining period preceded by a 20-week training period and an even longer detraining period (30–32 weeks) [123].

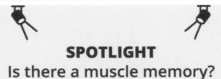

SPOTLIGHT
Is there a muscle memory?
· ·

The premiere theory used to explain muscle memory at the cellular level is that the increase in myonuclei during resistance training persists for a period of "detraining." This is a reasonable theory because the nuclei of muscle fibers are thought to have a long lifespan. If the previous training period resulted in more nuclei, the content of myonuclei will be maintained even after an extended period of detraining.

The same reasoning has been proposed in relation to doping and whether a two-year suspension is too short to make the positive effects of the previous doping episode disappear. It is indeed known that anabolic steroids can have a positive effect on myonuclear density [124], and a recent study demonstrated that muscle fibers from former steroid users had persistently higher myonuclei density and DNA-to-cytoplasm ratio four years after steroid discontinuation, which may indicate improved retraining ability [125]. However, several studies have indicated that muscle adaptations do not occur more rapidly during a training period that is performed after a long rest. The longevity of myonuclei is also questioned by research that reports a loss of myonuclei during detraining [126]. In one of the most systematic and recent reviews on this topic, the concept of skeletal muscle memory was questioned, at least when assuming the permanence of myonuclei [127].

Another possibility is that training leads to epigenetic changes that persist for a long time and positively influence the molecular response to exercise. In a relatively recent study, epigenetic changes were observed for the first time in humans after a previous period of muscle hypertrophy [128]. It was reported that the increase in muscle mass was greater during the retraining period than during the initial training period, and this may be related to the fact that DNA methylation was maintained during retraining, which then influenced gene expression during retraining 7 weeks later. These results are at odds with a study from the Karolinska Institutet in Stockholm, which showed that the pattern of gene expression after a single cycling training session was very comparable between an untrained and a previously trained leg [129]. Thus, the effect could be different between endurance and resistance training.

It should be emphasized that a somewhat simpler explanation for muscle memory is the habit of training and being able to perform various exercises with good form and effect. A person with previous training experience has probably learned the technique for a large number of exercises and is used to maximum intensities and large training volumes. In such a scenario, it is not surprising that getting fit again goes faster.

REGULATION OF PROTEIN BREAKDOWN

There are three main systems that regulate protein breakdown in skeletal muscle. These are the ubiquitin–proteasome pathway (UPP), autophagy, and the calpain–calcium–cysteine protease pathway [130]. UPP is the best characterized system and has been shown to be important for protein degradation in several cell types. The UPP system breaks down proteins tagged with ubiquitin for degradation. However, the UPP system cannot degrade intact myofibrils by itself. The calpain system is thought to be important for the degradation of sarcomere proteins.

The autophagy system interacts with the other systems and with cell lysosomes in the degradation of a variety of intracellular components such as membrane proteins, various types of transporters, ion channels, and receptors. Thus, all three systems interact in a coordinated response to facilitate adequate protein turnover during resistance training.

In the context of resistance training, protein breakdown is a necessary process to enable effective skeletal muscle remodeling. During periods of excessive muscular loading and during periods of inadequate recovery and/or nutrition, protein breakdown can be stimulated, resulting in a negative protein balance that leads to a net loss of muscle mass.

SUMMARY OF ESTABLISHED AND EMERGING MECHANISMS

Recently, an authoritative review paper on the mechanisms of muscle hypertrophy was published, involving many respected authors in the field [56]. This review highlights the mechanisms previously described in terms of the key factors involved in skeletal muscle hypertrophy induced by mechanical overload:

- **mTORC1 signaling:** the mTORC1 complex phosphorylates downstream targets involved in translation initiation and elongation, promoting muscle protein synthesis. Mechanical overload activates mTORC1 through mechanotransduction mechanisms such as increased diacylglycerol kinase activity/ PA and dissociation of TSC2 from lysosomes.

- **Ribosome biogenesis:** mechanical overload increases ribosomal RNA and total RNA content, expanding translational capacity through ribosome biogenesis. This precedes measurable hypertrophy and correlates with the extent of growth.

- **Satellite cells:** Satellite cells proliferate, differentiate, and fuse with myofibers in response to mechanical overload, contributing to the formation of new myonuclei. This process appears to be important for optimizing hypertrophy, especially during prolonged loading.

The authors also discussed other potential mechanisms that may be of interest, including the involvement of genetic variants, DNA methylation changes, extracellular matrix remodeling, angiogenesis, microRNAs, sex hormone signaling, prostaglandin signaling, β–adrenergic signaling, and more. Several emerging mechanisms were proposed that may regulate overload–induced hypertrophy, including mitochondrial biogenesis, metabolic adaptations, muscle circadian rhythms, microtubule dynamics, and gut microbiota.

In summary, the authors propose that skeletal muscle hypertrophy relies on the coordinated activity of multiple cellular and molecular mechanisms rather than a single dominant pathway (Fig. 7.4).

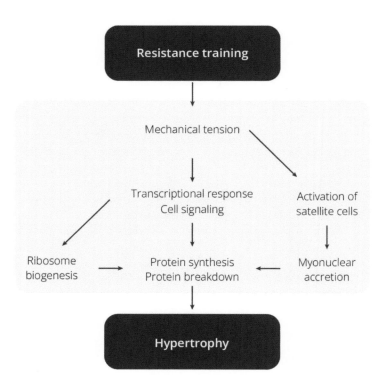

Figure 7.4.
Summary of the main mechanisms regulating muscle hypertrophy during resistance training.

SUMMARY

- Stimuli coupled with muscle hypertrophy include mechanical stress, metabolic stress, calcium signaling, free radicals, muscle fiber stretch, satellite cell activation, hormone release and growth factors, muscle damage, and cell swelling.

- A single bout of resistance training results in a variety of molecular responses that regulate gene and protein expression and coordinate the balance between protein synthesis and degradation.

- The molecular response to resistance training is complex and involves events throughout the chain from DNA to gene expression (mRNA) to protein translation in the ribosomes.

- Non–genetic structural changes in DNA can affect gene expression, which is referred to as epigenetics.

- Resistance training alters the expression of genes involved in a variety of functions, including cell growth, inflammation, and protein degradation.

- Increased translation rate of mRNA into protein (translation efficiency) is important for the rapid increase in protein synthesis that occurs after resistance training.

- Translation of mRNA into protein involves three steps: initiation, elongation, and termination. Of particular importance is the initiation step, which is coordinated by a protein complex called mTOR (mechanistic target of rapamycin).

- mTOR integrates signals derived from mechanical stimuli, energy status, and nutrients (mainly amino acids) to coordinate signaling cascades that promote increased protein synthesis.

- Over time, the new formation and improved function of ribosomes are also required for protein synthesis to continue to increase as the muscle grows. This process is called ribosome biogenesis.

- The "myonuclear domain theory" is based on the notion that the ratio between fiber volume and the number of nuclei should be relatively constant to maintain the capacity for transcription and protein synthesis.

- It is believed that satellite cells fuse with the muscle fiber during long-term training and become mature myonuclei. Thus, resistance training can increase the number of nuclei in the muscle fiber.

- It has been suggested that the increase in myonuclei contributes to a so-called "muscle memory" effect. However, scientific support for this theory is still rather weak.

- Three main systems regulate protein degradation in skeletal muscle: the ubiquitin-proteasome pathway (UPP), autophagy, and the calpain-calcium-cysteine protease pathway.

08

METABOLIC AND HORMONAL ADAPTATIONS

Resistance training affects the metabolism of the entire body, including skeletal muscle. During heavy resistance training, working muscles can have energy turnovers 200 times greater than at rest. The increased energy demand results from the need for ATP for the muscle contraction process. Various hormones are also released to support the increased energy metabolism and to maintain blood glucose levels. After prolonged training, metabolic adaptations have taken place that better equip the body for future exertion. This chapter discusses both acute and long–term metabolic and hormonal adaptations to resistance training.

ACUTE METABOLIC RESPONSE TO RESISTANCE TRAINING

As mentioned in Chapter 2, the acute metabolic response to resistance training is influenced by the design of the training session. A program with high loads, few repetitions, and long rest periods will primarily stress the anaerobic energy systems, i.e., the phosphocreatine system and the breakdown of muscle glycogen (glycolysis). In contrast, a program with many repetitions performed to failure and short rest periods will stress both the anaerobic and aerobic systems.

Estimation of energy expenditure during physical work is usually done by measuring oxygen uptake. Although this method is not usually used in resistance training, there are some published studies that have examined this area. Interestingly, traditional resistance training that targets the larger muscle groups of the lower limbs results in oxygen consumption of approximately 50–60% of maximal oxygen uptake, even with relatively long periods of rest between sets [131]. This level of oxygen consumption is surprisingly high to many and suggests that it is possible to achieve the recommended moderate intensity for aerobic physical activity through resistance training alone [132].

After 30 minutes of leg press resistance training (4 sets × 6–12 repetitions), the levels of all dominant energy substrates in muscle decrease to varying degrees (ATP, phosphocreatine, glycogen, and triglycerides). In addition, plasma lactate levels can increase up to 12 mmol/liter during portions of the training session [133]. Thus, during a typical resistance training program, all energy systems are active to varying degrees, even though the anaerobic systems dominate during the actual lifting.

With respect to specific muscle fiber types, glycogen levels decrease during resistance training in both type 1 and type 2 fibers. At an intensity equivalent to 70% of 1RM, glycogen depletion is greater in type 2 fibers than in type 1 fibers [134].

Whether the metabolic stress associated with resistance training is an important stimulus for muscle adaptation to resistance training is not fully understood. However, as discussed in Chapter 7, several of the signaling pathways triggered by increased energetic stress (e.g., calcium signaling, PGC1–α, and AMPK) may play a role in regulating muscle protein turnover, likely in both positive and negative ways, depending on circumstances.

LONG–TERM ADAPTATIONS

Capillaries

The view of longer–term metabolic adaptations to resistance training has changed to some extent in recent years, not least in terms of how resistance training promotes the proliferation of new capillaries around muscle fibers (angiogenesis). In the 1970s, it was found that the number of capillaries can increase with endurance training. Resistance training was thought to decrease capillary density because fiber area increased while the number of capillaries did not change. Thus, the number of capillaries per fiber was constant, while the number of capillaries per fiber area decreased. It could be argued that the latter metric is more relevant because the supply of oxygen and other substrates to the fibers may be compromised when the capillary density is lower.

More recently, however, an increasing number of training studies in both young and old people have shown that capillarization can also increase with resistance training [135,136]. This is particularly true for the number of capillaries per fiber, with the important consequence that capillary density remains constant even though the fiber has increased in size.

The extent to which capillary formation occurs during resistance training likely depends on the type of resistance training performed. A larger total training volume generated by more sets and/or repetitions is more likely to trigger capillarization than a heavy–weight, low–volume workout because important stimuli for angiogenesis, such as increased blood flow, shear stress, stretching of muscle fibers, and reduced oxygen supply, increase with such training. Increasing the number of capillaries increases the ability to maintain muscle blood flow, substrate supply, and delivery of amino acids, which are the building blocks for protein synthesis.

There is also some evidence that capillarization is important for optimal satellite cell function. Individuals with higher capillary density show greater activation of satellite cells during resistance training [137], and satellite cell function generally appears to be related to the anatomical distance between satellite cells and blood vessels [138]. Interestingly, in a study of older people, those with the largest capillary network around muscle fibers responded better to resistance training, as expressed by an increase in muscle mass, than those with a smaller network [139]. However, this was not seen in younger people [140].

A CLOSER LOOK: Immunohistochemistry

Immunohistochemistry on muscle tissue is used in the context of resistance training to study, for example, the size of fibers, fiber types, capillaries, the number of nuclei and satellite cells, or the presence of specific proteins or immune cells. Instead of using a protein homogenate (as in Western blotting), very thin cross–sections of the muscle sample are cut and then collected on a slide. Antibodies and fluorescence can be used to photograph the sections and analyze the images showing the stained proteins. A minced muscle biopsy that has been treated with chemicals in a test tube cannot be used for this purpose. An example of a muscle section where immunohistochemistry has been applied can be found in Figure 8.1.

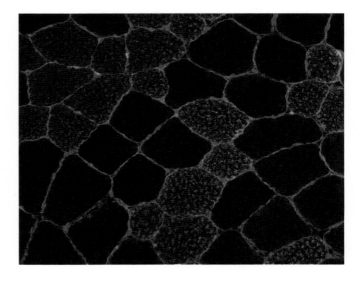

Figure 8.1.
Cross–section of a muscle biopsy stained and photographed with specific antibodies for cell membranes (red), type 1 fibers (green), nuclei (blue), and capillaries (white). This technique is called immunohistochemistry.

Mitochondria

Just over a dozen studies have examined how mitochondrial content is affected by resistance training. Most commonly, the activity of the enzyme citrate synthase has been used as a marker of mitochondrial content because this enzyme correlates well with the number of mitochondria in muscle. Most studies have shown that mitochondrial content remains unchanged after resistance training (usually after 10–12 weeks of training). Since most resistance training studies are associated with an increase in fiber area, this means that mitochondrial density (mitochondrial content per fiber area) decreases.

However, research results are not unanimous, as there are studies that also report an increase in mitochondrial content [141]. Although there are training modes that are more effective than resistance training in increasing mitochondrial density, the outcome ultimately depends on the specific design of the program. For example, low–load, high–volume resistance training could result in an increase in mitochondrial content.

More recently, mitochondrial function has also been studied by measuring mitochondrial respiratory capacity. Again, research is conflicting [142,143], and results depend on the training status of the subjects, the intensity of the training, and the timing of the measurement in relation to the completion of training.

Metabolic enzyme levels

Resistance training generally has a rather small effect on various enzymes involved in aerobic and anaerobic energy metabolism. Aerobic enzymes studied include SDH, citrate synthase, and beta– HAD. While these enzymes are generally unchanged during resistance training, bodybuilders who frequently perform many sets and repetitions may have elevated levels of some of these aerobic enzymes [133].

One might spontaneously assume that resistance training would instead increase levels of anaerobic enzymes. Phosphofructokinase, lactate dehydrogenase, myokinase, and creatine kinase have been studied here. Although a few studies have shown significant changes, overall the data suggest that resistance training has little effect on anaerobic enzyme levels [133].

Glycogen

A consistent finding in the literature is that muscle glycogen storage increases with resistance training, just as it does with endurance training. Thus, after a period of resistance training, the size of glycogen stores increases compared to before the training period. This increase can be about 20% after 5 weeks of resistance training and can increase even more after combined strength and endurance training [61].

HORMONAL ADAPTATIONS

Hormones are transported through the blood to all tissues but act mainly on target cells that have specific receptors that can bind these hormones. These receptors may decrease in number when chronically exposed to high levels of hormones or increase when exposed to low levels. After the hormone is bound to the receptor, cell activity is influenced by several different mechanisms:

- ➲ Effects on membrane transport mechanisms
- ➲ Stimulation of DNA in the nucleus, which initiates the synthesis of a specific protein
- ➲ Activation of secondary messengers in the cell

In the context of resistance training, stimulation of DNA in the nucleus and activation of secondary messengers are important mechanisms. Steroid hormones readily diffuse across the cell membrane where they bind to a protein receptor in the cytoplasm. This steroid receptor complex enters the nucleus and binds to specific proteins associated with DNA, which contains the codes for protein synthesis. This initiates the steps that lead to the synthesis of specific mRNAs. The mRNAs then transport the code from the nucleus to the cytoplasm, where the specific proteins are synthesized in the ribosomes.

Because of their size or charge, some hormones cannot cross the cell membrane. These hormones exert their effects by binding to a receptor on the membrane surface, which activates a G protein located in the membrane. The G protein is thus the link between the outside and the inside of the cell.

Growth hormone (GH)

GH is produced in the pituitary gland. The release of the hormone influences the growth of all tissues through local growth factors such as insulin–like growth factors (IGF). GH and IGF stimulate tissue uptake of amino acids, bone growth, and synthesis of new proteins. GH spares plasma glucose by having the opposite effect of insulin. GH also increases the synthesis of glucose in the liver (gluconeogenesis) and the mobilization of fatty acids from adipose tissue.

GH increases during physical work, which facilitates the release of glucose into the blood plasma. Normally, the release of GH is highest at night. The release of GH increases during resistance training. However, while GH may undoubtedly have anabolic effects on various cells, including muscle fibers, the exercise–induced release of GH and IGF does not appear to be critical for the increased muscle protein synthesis seen acutely after exercise. The importance of circulating hormones to muscle hypertrophy was discussed in more detail in Chapter 7.

Insulin

Insulin is secreted by the beta cells of the pancreas. Insulin is the most important hormone in the absorption phase when nutrients enter the bloodstream. Insulin stimulates tissue absorption of glucose and amino acids. Insulin also facilitates the process by which blood glucose passes through the cell membrane via various glucose transporters. Insulin secretion is controlled by plasma glucose levels, blood amino acid concentrations, sympathetic and parasympathetic nervous system stimulation, and levels of other hormones. Insulin is considered an anabolic hormone and acts primarily by inhibiting protein breakdown. However, insulin secretion is generally inhibited during resistance training and is not considered an important factor in regulating protein turnover after resistance training [144].

Insulin–Like Growth Factor (IGF)

IGF is one of the most studied anabolic hormones in the body. IGF–1 is a peptide hormone structurally similar to insulin, hence the name. IGF–1 responds to mechanical stress and has been associated with hypertrophy in several different models [145]. However, it has been reported that muscle hypertrophy is intact even when the receptor for IGF–1 is blocked [103]. Moreover, the increase in IGF–1 does not correlate with hypertrophy [146], and there is no benefit to hypertrophy when IGF–1 levels are increased via exercise before resistance training [102]. Thus, most researchers agree that the exercise–induced increase in protein synthesis is independent of IGF–1.

Sex hormones

The secretion of testosterone is controlled by negative feedback mechanisms from the pituitary and hypothalamus. Testosterone has both anabolic and androgenic effects. Testosterone is important for muscular development in boys during the pubertal growth phase and for the development of male sex characteristics. The female sex hormone estrogen stimulates breast growth, fat storage, and other female sex characteristics. The importance of sex hormones in explaining biological sex differences in resistance training is discussed in more detail in Chapter 17.

Testosterone undoubtedly has anabolic effects on skeletal muscle. Free testosterone that is not bound to transport proteins in the blood binds to androgen receptors. Testosterone is then transported to the nucleus, where it can interact with the cell's DNA. Testosterone can affect protein synthesis and degradation as well as satellite cell function. Although testosterone levels increase during acute exercise, it is now agreed that testosterone is not a crucial regulator of muscle hypertrophy during resistance training (see Chapter 7). Nevertheless, supraphysiological doses of testosterone can have marked effects on muscle mass [147]. Testosterone is also largely responsible for the differences in muscle mass between males and females that manifest during puberty [148].

Cytokines

During resistance training, hormone–like cytokines are produced locally in skeletal muscle. The cytokines produced in muscle are usually referred to as "myokines". Many of these myokines have been associated with acute and chronic inflammation in various disease states. However, in healthy muscle, these myokines are involved in a variety of physiological processes thought to be important in training adaptations, including angiogenesis, hypertrophy, inflammatory processes, and regulation of extracellular matrix composition [149].

Some of the best described myokines are interleukin–6 and TNF–α. Myostatin is also often included in the group of myokines. The importance of myostatin in muscle hypertrophy was described in Chapter 7. What these myokines have in common is that they can affect important signaling pathways involved in the regulation of muscle protein turnover during resistance training. This may be one of the reasons why interventions that suppress inflammation in young healthy individuals have a negative effect on hypertrophy (see Chapter 14), whereas the opposite may be true in older individuals with low–grade chronic inflammation [150].

SUMMARY

- Resistance training affects both the aerobic and anaerobic energy systems, with the design of the training program ultimately determining the acute metabolic response to exercise.

- During a set of high-intensity resistance training, phosphocreatine and muscle glycogen are the major energy substrates for ATP production.

- The importance of acute metabolic stress for long-term muscle adaptation to resistance training has not been fully elucidated.

- Resistance training can lead to the formation of new capillaries, which means that capillary density is kept constant.

- New research suggests that the capillary network may be important for the long-term ability to build muscle mass, at least in older people.

- Most resistance training studies have found unchanged mitochondrial content, and thus lower mitochondrial density, when fiber cross-sectional area increases.

- Resistance training is generally associated with little or no change in aerobic and anaerobic enzyme levels.

- The ability to store glycogen in muscle increases with resistance training.

- Resistance training results in increased secretion of growth hormone, IGF-1, and testosterone, while insulin secretion is inhibited.

- The exercise-induced change in the levels of these hormones appears to be of little importance for long-term training adaptation.

- Resistance training leads to increased production of hormone-like cytokines in muscles called myokines. Several of these myokines, such as IL-6 and TNF-α, may affect important signaling pathways involved in the regulation of muscle protein turnover during resistance training.

CHAPTER 09

MUSCLE ARCHITECTURE, BONE, AND ELASTIC COMPONENTS

Although maximum force is determined in large part by muscle size, fiber type composition, and neural activation, muscle architecture and extracellular matrix composition can also influence the ability to generate force. In this chapter, we will examine how these factors adapt to resistance training.

MUSCLE ARCHITECTURE

During the process of muscle hypertrophy, more sarcomeres are added parallel to each other, resulting in an increase in fiber cross-sectional area. However, muscle hypertrophy can also occur by the addition of sarcomeres in series, resulting in longitudinal growth of the fascicles. Typically, the pennation angle (the fiber direction relative to the anatomic direction from origin to attachment) also increases. As discussed in Chapter 3, a larger pennation angle has a positive effect on muscle force development because it allows more sarcomeres to be packed into the same anatomical cross-section. This increases the physiological cross-section of the muscle compared to the anatomical cross-section.

However, it should be noted that the shortening force of the muscle acts in the anatomical direction from origin to attachment. Therefore, there is a limit beyond which a greater pennation angle is no longer favorable for force production. Force increases with increasing pennation angle up to an angle of 45°. A pennation angle beyond this limit would be too perpendicular to the pulling direction to produce optimal force. Since most skeletal muscles are far from this threshold, a greater pennation angle typically results in a greater potential for force development in most muscles. However, the importance of pennation angle to muscle function is controversial and difficult to verify directly. Some have argued that this is a packing strategy that allows short fibers to be packed into a limited volume without any functional significance [151].

A logical follow-up question is: are there advantages to having the fascicles run in the anatomical direction of the muscle? The answer is yes, because such an arrangement results in greater shortening of the muscle for a given force output. Since each sarcomere can only be shortened to a certain degree, the overall shortening of the muscle is greater when more sarcomeres are connected in series than in a more pennate muscle. Thus, a muscle with many sarcomeres in series (long fascicles) is faster than a pennate muscle. This is consistent with the typical appearance of muscles in the body. Large muscles that usually generate high forces, such as the gluteus maximus, are relatively pennate. In contrast, the fascicles of the hamstring muscles are more longitudinal because they must shorten considerably to flex the knee joint, for example, during a sprint.

A CLOSER LOOK: Ultrasound

. . . .

Ultrasound is used to study the architecture of muscles and fascicles (Fig. 9.1). The factors measured in resistance training studies are usually muscle thickness, pennation angle, and fascicle length. Ultrasound is a relatively simple and inexpensive method, but it requires specialized equipment, knowledge, and experience. Also, the precision and reproducibility are poorer than in some other imaging modalities, and it is difficult to measure the size or volume of deep-lying muscles. However, ultrasound is still the best option for measuring the pennation angle and fascicle length.

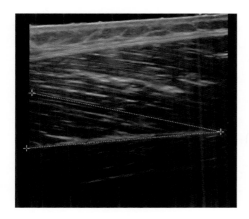

Figure 9.1.
Ultrasound image of the skeletal muscle. The image shows how the pennation angle and fascicle length (truncated in the image) can be identified by ultrasound.

Adaptations to resistance training

Muscle contraction results in immediate shortening of fibers. Based on ultrasound measurements, it has been reported that the fascicles in the calf muscle (gastrocnemius) are shortened by 35–50% during a maximal contraction at optimal ankle angle [12]. This severe shortening of the fibers means that there is a large and immediate increase in the angle of the fibers. However, how much the fibers are shortened during a given maximal contraction depends on the actual joint angle, moment arm, and tendon stiffness.

A longer-term increase in pennation angle and fascicle length may parallel and coincide with the expected increase in muscle cross-sectional area during resistance training. A Danish study conducted two decades ago clearly showed that the pennation angle increased with resistance training, although there were individual differences [152]. In this study, the vastus lateralis pennation angle increased from 8 to 11° after 14 weeks of resistance training for knee extensors. The following figure shows the results of a 35-day resistance training study that used a flywheel ergometer to provide both concentric and eccentric resistance (Fig. 9.2). As you can see from the figure, the structural changes in the muscle can occur quite quickly [153].

Figure 9.2.
Changes in muscle architecture (fascicle length, pennation angle, and muscle cross-sectional area) during 35 days of resistance training for knee extensors. Based on data from Seyennes et al. 2007. The complete reference can be found in the Figure references section at the end of the book.

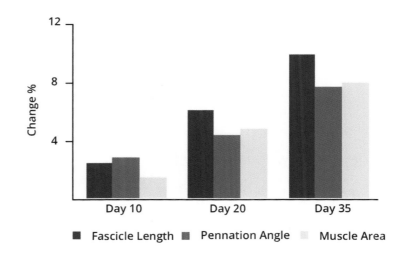

SPOTLIGHT
Can the type of muscle action used during resistance training affect architectural adaptations?

· ·

In both young and older people, the type of muscle action used during training can affect muscle architecture. Both concentric and eccentric training can lead to an increase in muscle volume [154], but this hypertrophy may be achieved in part by different mechanisms. Although conclusive evidence is lacking, concentric training is thought to result in an increase in pennation angle with little change in fascicle length, whereas eccentric training results in a greater increase in fascicle length and less pronounced changes in pennation angle. This means that the addition of sarcomeres can occur in parallel or in series, and that the result may depend on the type of muscle action used in the training program. Thus, concentric resistance training leads to muscle growth through the parallel addition of sarcomeres, while eccentric training, at least to a greater extent than concentric training, leads to hypertrophy through the addition of sarcomeres in series (Fig. 9.3).

Sarcomeres in series

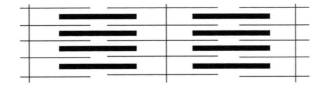

Figure 9.3.
Sarcomeres can be added in series or in parallel after resistance training.

Sarcomeres in parallel

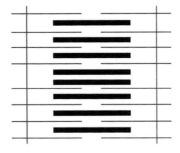

Do changes in fiber length contribute to hypertrophy?

In addition to affecting muscle force production, changes in fiber length may also impact whole–muscle cross–sectional area. Indeed, some evidence suggests that an increase in fiber length may occur and play an important role in chronic mechanical overload. Calculations suggest that a 13% increase in fiber length alone could increase the cross–sectional area of the muscle and the number of fibers per cross–section by over 50% [155]. This is because longer fibers are packed and stacked more densely to occupy a larger cross–sectional area.

Rapid changes in length have been observed to occur within a few days of the onset of overload before greater fiber thickening occurs. Thus, it is possible that length changes contribute significantly to the rapid muscle growth observed in overload models before the cross–sectional area increases significantly. Therefore, some models may have overlooked fiber length as an important variable affecting muscle hypertrophy.

THE ELASTIC COMPONENTS

Tendons and connective tissue

Tendons and connective tissue differ from muscle tissue in many ways. The tissue is composed of collagen fibers and contains relatively small amounts of cells (mainly fibroblasts) intermingled with collagen fibers, matrix proteins (mainly collagen type 1), glycoproteins, and glycosaminoglycans. For a long time, research on tendon physiology was dominated by studies investigating biomechanical aspects of tendon function, tendon surgery, and rehabilitation of tendon injuries. Tendon tissue is more difficult to study than skeletal muscle, and tendons were thought to have modest protein turnover.

More recently, however, tendon tissue has been shown to respond markedly to both unloading and exercise, and protein turnover is much higher than previously thought. Whereas the protein turnover of skeletal muscle is about 1–2% per day, the turnover of tendons is about half of that [156]. It is worth noting, however, that although much of the tendon is dynamic and responds to external stressors, there is collagen in the central parts of the tendon that is thought to have no turnover at all in adulthood [157].

Tendons have varying degrees of elasticity, usually referred to as stiffness. The degree of stiffness affects how much energy can be stored and released during work. For example, in the Achilles tendon, about 5% elongation occurs during maximal isometric contraction. The properties of the tendon, not least its stiffness, are of great importance for the transmission of force from the muscle to the bone to which the tendon attaches. The degree of stiffness is correlated with muscle strength, with greater stiffness being associated with a greater ability to develop force.

The stiffness of the tendon is determined by its structural and architectural characteristics. There are relatively large differences between tendons of different muscle groups. Stiffness can also significantly affect the work economy during endurance–oriented activities. This is illustrated by the correlation between tendon stiffness and running economy in endurance athletes (see Chapter 15).

Extracellular matrix proteins

The extracellular matrix of muscle also contains a network of cytoskeletal proteins important for force transmission in muscle, both along the muscle fibers and from the center of the fibers outward (laterally). While the cross–bridge cycle with myosin and actin is responsible for producing mechanical tension, the force generated must be transmitted from the fibers to the connective tissue and tendon, which in turn connects the muscle to the bone. Important components in this system are proteins within the muscle fibers, such as titin, nebulin, alpha–actinin, and dystrophin, but also extracellular proteins such as costameres, the various collagen proteins and the dystrophin–associated glycoprotein complex [158].

Adaptation to resistance training

Connective tissue makes up about 10% of muscle volume. Although this number appears to be fairly constant regardless of training status [159], tendon and the entire extracellular matrix complex respond to resistance training [160]. In one of the first studies to measure collagen protein synthesis in humans, the duration of the increase in protein synthesis in response to exercise was found to be comparable to protein synthesis in skeletal muscle [161]. The peak in protein synthesis occurred 24 hours after training and was still slightly increased after 72 hours. However, the magnitude of the increase was less in tendon (1.7–fold) than in muscle (2.8–fold). In general, resistance training leads to both increases in tendon size and stiffness, with the effect on stiffness being slightly greater than the effect on cross–sectional area. Loads above 70% of 1RM appear to be required for these tendon adaptations to occur, whereas the choice of muscle action appears to be less important [162].

Increasing tendon stiffness through resistance training means that more force is required to stretch the elastic components. This, in turn, allows for a faster increase in the force curve during a maximal contraction (i.e., a higher rate of force development). Remodeling of tendon structure involves the process of "cross–linking," in which the anchors present between collagen filaments are affected by training.

Different training programs have been shown to affect tendon and extracellular matrix stiffness in different ways. Heavy resistance training combined with explosive exercises and plyometric jumps results in increased cross–linking, increased collagen content, and increased stiffness in the extracellular matrix complex. This means that force transfer from muscle to bone is faster, which is important for muscle strength and speed [163].

In contrast, resistance training with slower movement speeds, such as sustained isometric contractions or slow eccentric actions, results in less cross–linking in the part of the muscle closest to the tendon (myotendinous junction). The reduced stiffness at the muscle–tendon junction leads to better resistance to large forces, so the risk of injury is likely to decrease with this type of training [163].

BONE TISSUE

Bone tissue is composed of both cells and extracellular matrix. The main cell types are osteoblasts, osteoclasts, and osteocytes. Osteoblasts produce the bone substance. Osteocytes are produced by osteoblasts and maintain bone substance, while osteoclasts break down bone. The bone matrix is largely composed of inorganic salts, mainly calcium phosphate. In addition, collagen fibers are embedded in the bone tissue, which helps the bone withstand high tensile forces.

To positively affect bone turnover, the mechanical load during resistance training should exceed the load from daily physical activity. Therefore, swimming, cycling, and walking have limited effects on bone health [164]. For resistance training, the best effects have been observed when high loads are used (about 80% of 1RM), when exercise is performed at least twice per week, and when large muscle groups are used, including those involving the hip and spine [165].

The mechanical stress that occurs during resistance training has a positive effect on osteocytes and osteoblasts. These cells sense the mechanical stress and increase bone synthesis [166]. The response to exercise is greatest in the areas of the bone where the mechanical stress was greatest. Similar to the connective tissue response, bone osteocytes quickly become insensitive to mechanical stimulation [167]. Therefore, short training sessions with repeated mechanical stimulation are more effective in promoting bone adaptation than when the appropriate volume of training is performed on a single occasion [168].

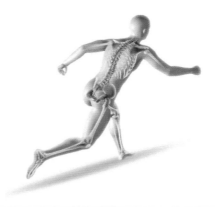

SUMMARY

- Muscle hypertrophy can occur by both parallel and serial addition of sarcomeres.

- Parallel addition of sarcomeres results in an increase in pennation angle and radial growth of fascicles, whereas serial addition of sarcomeres results in an increase in fascicle length (longitudinal growth of fascicles).

- The force a muscle can generate generally increases with increasing pennation angle.

- Large fascicle lengths, i.e., many sarcomeres in series, are beneficial for the speed of contraction (the change in muscle length for a given force).

- Concentric exercise leads to an increase in pennation angle with relatively little change in fascicle length, whereas eccentric training can lead to an increase in fascicle length to a greater extent than concentric training.

- Changes in muscle fiber length can contribute to muscle hypertrophy.

- The biochemical composition of tendon and connective tissue differs from that of skeletal muscle, where various collagens are an important component of tendon and connective tissue. This contributes to high tensile strength.

- Increased stiffness of tendon and connective tissue is beneficial for force transfer from muscle to bone.

- Although the cross-bridge cycle with myosin and actin produces the mechanical force, the force must be transmitted from the fibers to the connective tissue and tendon, which in turn connect the muscle to the bone.

- The extracellular matrix of the muscle therefore also contains a network of cytoskeletal proteins, which are of great importance for this force transmission.

- The stiffness of the tendon increases with resistance training, meaning that more force is required to stretch the elastic components. This means that rapid force production (rate of force development) is improved.

- Bone turnover is controlled by the activity of bone cells (osteoclasts, osteoblasts, and osteocytes).

- Short, repetitive mechanical loads are more effective for bone adaptation than when the same volume of training is performed on a single occasion.

PART 3

DETERMINANTS OF RESISTANCE TRAINING OUTCOMES

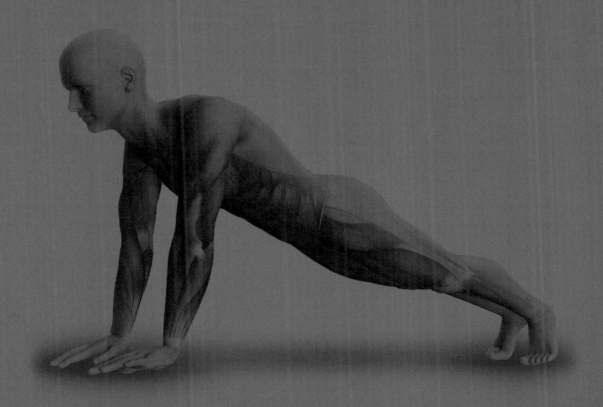

CHAPTER 10

TRAINING VARIABLES AND PROGRAM DESIGN

There are many factors to consider when designing a resistance training program – and it can be challenging. Goals vary from person to person, the individual response is large, and there are so many training variables that can be manipulated. Changing one variable directly or indirectly affects several other variables. In this chapter, we will discuss some of the most important training variables that affect resistance training adaptations.

GENERAL TRAINING PRINCIPLES

Perhaps the most fundamental training principle is the principle of **overload**. Overload means that a system or tissue must be stressed to a reasonably high level for a training effect to occur. The tissue or system then responds by gradually adapting to this overload. Overload is not only achieved by increasing the intensity (load) of training. It is also possible to create an overload by, for example, changing the:

- ➲ total volume (number of sets and reps)
- ➲ frequency of training
- ➲ selection of exercises
- ➲ degree of effort (how close to failure)
- ➲ range of motion
- ➲ form/technique
- ➲ internal vs. external focus

The principle of **reversibility** means that the training effects obtained by progressive overload are reversible and gradually decline when the stimuli decrease or stop. The extent of reversibility may depend on training status. In untrained subjects who increased muscle strength and hypertrophy during 3 months of training, most of these adaptations (with the exception of peak power in high–velocity contractions) had reverted to pretraining levels after a 3–month break in training [76]. Trained strength athletes, however, may see a decrease in muscle function and muscle fiber size after only 2 weeks of detraining [169].

The principle of **specificity** means that the training effect is specific to the exercise performed, the muscles involved, the range of motion, the joint angle, the speed of contraction, and the type of muscle contraction. A good example is that strength improvements are usually greatest when the test closely matches the training exercise. If you compare dynamic and isometric training, the gains are greatest for the exercise type that was trained [170].

TRAINING VARIABLES

Textbooks usually say that the training result depends on the intensity, duration, and frequency of training. If you multiply these factors, you get the total training volume. In the context of resistance training, the duration of the workout is of little interest because it is largely determined by the rest period between sets and exercises. Instead, the number of sets and repetitions determines the training volume. Training volume is therefore often defined as the number of sets × repetitions × training frequency. It is also common to add intensity (the load lifted) as an additional factor, since higher intensity leads to more work done when the other factors are constant. Training volume and frequency are closely related, as an increase in training frequency often leads to a higher weekly training volume.

Training volume

There is a dose–dependent relationship between training volume and the acute anabolic response to exercise. Multiple sets of resistance training stimulate muscle protein synthesis more than one set [171]. However, the acute response and subsequent long–term training adaptation are not necessarily correlated. We must therefore turn to actual training studies to uncover the relationship between training volume and muscular adaptations.

One meta–analysis found that there was a dose–dependent relationship between training volume and muscle hypertrophy, at least up to 10 sets per muscle group per week [172], although it should be noted that the vast majority of studies in this meta–analysis examined untrained subjects. A study of strength–trained men compared three different training volumes (1, 3, or 5 sets per exercise) with a matched training frequency (3 sessions per week for 8 weeks). The results confirmed that there was a dose–dependent correlation between training volume and muscle hypertrophy [173].

Interestingly, training volume was not as important for the development of strength in this meta–analysis. This may be in part because intensity (load) is an important factor in strength gains, and choosing a high load often means fewer repetitions and a relatively limited number of sets, given the need for rest and maximal effort. Thus, greater volumes of resistance training are likely to result in greater strength gains up to a certain point, e.g., 2–3 sets per exercise stimulate greater strength gains than 1 set per exercise, but after that, it is questionable whether further increases in dose would result in greater gains [174].

In terms of individual responsiveness to training volume, a recent study provided new insights by subjecting untrained individuals to moderate– and low–volume contralateral resistance training for 12 weeks [175]. Of 34 participants, thirteen showed a clear benefit of increased volume on muscle hypertrophy and sixteen showed a clear benefit on muscle strength gains. This shows that everyone responds individually to increased training volume, meaning that some seem to benefit more than others. Interestingly, the authors found that ribosomal biogenesis (discussed in Chapter 7 as an important hypertrophy mechanism) regulates the dose–response relationship between training volume and muscle hypertrophy.

Training Frequency

As mentioned in Chapter 4, muscle protein synthesis is increased for 24–72 hours after acute resistance exercise. On this basis, it could be hypothesized that two or three exercise sessions per week should provide a sustained increase in protein synthesis, which should be beneficial for muscle hypertrophy.

Surprisingly, the correlation between training frequency and training outcome is rather weak. One meta–analysis found that training frequency was of little importance for muscle hypertrophy when matching for training volume [176]. However, another meta–analysis found that muscle hypertrophy is somewhat improved at 2 and 3 sessions per week compared with one session per week, even when the total training volume is the same [177]. Overall, it appears that total training volume is more important than training frequency, at least if training occurs once per week or more. However, increasing the training frequency is a practical way to increase the total training volume. Thus, increased training frequency can indirectly promote muscle hypertrophy by promoting a higher training volume.

The importance of training frequency in increasing maximal strength shows a similar pattern. Training frequency is important, but primarily because total training volume increases with increasing training frequency [178]. The marginal importance of training frequency during short–term training periods was further demonstrated in a study comparing exercise 5 times per week with training 3 or 2 times per week [179]. There was a surprisingly small effect of increased training frequency on both muscle size and 1RM strength, although the frequency of 5 times per week resulted in a higher total training volume than the other two frequencies.

Training frequency is likely to be of greater importance for strength development in young compared with older individuals and in trained compared with untrained individuals. The latter hypothesis is based on the anabolic response to acute exercise, in which the duration of the protein synthetic response decreases in the trained state. Therefore, there is more opportunity to increase protein turnover between training sessions through additional training. However, even in trained participants, no differences were found between groups in muscle growth or strength when comparing the volume–equivalent training frequency of 2 or 4 weekly sessions

[180]. Thus, training individual muscle groups 2 times per week seems to be a recommendation that can apply to both untrained and trained individuals.

Rest period between sets

In the old literature on resistance training, it is sometimes argued that rest periods between sets should be short if the goal is to maximize muscle hypertrophy, and long if the goal is maximal strength. The argument for this was that short rest periods increase the overall stress on the muscles and that both hormonal and metabolic responses are more pronounced with short rest periods. The research literature does not agree with this theory. It appears that rest periods are of little importance, especially for maximizing muscle hypertrophy [181]. In fact, long rest periods allow for recovery of strength between sets, which translates into better execution of the next set.

A relatively recent study reported that muscle hypertrophy was greater in trained subjects with 3 minutes of rest than with 1 minute of rest and this was explained by improved exercise performance that allowed for greater total training volume [182]. In addition, a shorter rest period between sets (1 minute versus 5 minutes) is associated with an attenuated protein synthetic response [183]. Thus, it appears that shortening the rest period between sets may attenuate the anabolic response, likely by attenuating key molecular signals that turn on muscle protein synthesis [183]. These acute results confirm studies reporting increased muscle hypertrophy with longer rest. It should be noted that the acute comparison of 1 vs. 5 minutes is quite extreme, and there is currently no consensus on the exact recovery time required to maximize the benefits of resistance training.

Optimal rest time likely depends on the type of exercise performed, the muscle groups involved, and overall training status. Multi–joint exercises such as Olympic weightlifting may require longer rest periods than stabilization exercises for small muscle groups. Indeed, long rests are preferable when heavy explosive lifts are to be performed. Phosphocreatine stores need several minutes to recover. Until this is done, it is impossible to perform at the same level as in the previous set.

Whether the nervous system also requires a rest period between sets to recover is unclear and may depend on the specific training program being performed [184]. Nevertheless, a long rest period allows for the recovery of phosphocreatine stores and the elimination of free phosphate ions and other molecules that interfere with the contractile machinery. Thus, if the development of maximal strength is the primary concern, relatively long rest periods (>2 minutes) should be used.

A disadvantage of longer rest periods is that the training session takes longer. From a practical standpoint, and especially for recreational athletes seeking health benefits, shorter rest periods are preferable because they allow additional exercises to be performed within the same time frame.

Intensity

In the context of resistance training, intensity is the load, weight, or resistance used in a particular exercise. Intensity is often expressed as a % of 1RM. When the exercise is performed to muscular exhaustion (near failure), it means that low intensity is associated with many repetitions, while high intensity means that only a few repetitions can be performed.

The view of the importance of intensity for muscle hypertrophy has changed significantly in recent years. For example, a review article published in 2010 claimed that intensity was the most important factor in stimulating muscle growth [185]. Several review articles published in recent years have instead cited training volume and degree of effort as the most important factors.

Why has the view of the importance of exercise intensity for muscle hypertrophy evolved? One reason is the earlier overemphasis, often repeated in textbooks, on repetition ranges suitable for different goals: Maximal strength, power, hypertrophy, and muscle endurance. Most people involved in resistance training will be familiar with these tables, which generally suggest 8–12 repetitions for "hypertrophy training." However, a thorough examination of the scientific literature reveals that these simplified tables do not have a solid evidence–based foundation.

The overemphasis on repetition ranges is based in part on a misunderstanding of Henneman's size principle, which points to the need for a more nuanced perspective. The size principle states that the small motor units are recruited first and then, with heavier loads, the larger motor units follow. It has been argued that training with light weights is ineffective because not all motor units are recruited and thus not all muscle fibers are stimulated to grow. However, the argument that recruitment is proportional to load applies mainly at rest. During fatigue, motor unit recruitment increases to compensate for muscle fatigue.

There is also a theory that when fatigue occurs, there is a rotation of the different motor units [186]. Thus, when muscles are exercised at a low load to near task failure, most fibers are recruited and stimulated, just as they are at higher exercise intensities. In support of this hypothesis, it has been reported that intensity has very little, if any, significance for the protein synthetic response when training is performed to failure [187].

Today we know that muscle hypertrophy can be achieved with a wide range of loads and repetitions. Training studies have convincingly shown that this is true for both trained and untrained individuals. When comparing a traditional resistance training program (80% of 1RM) to lighter loads equivalent to 30% of 1RM, these training programs result in identical muscle hypertrophy [188]. However, when training with lighter loads, it is important to approach failure to stimulate all muscle fibers.

The number of repetitions that can be performed at a certain load depends, in part, on the specific exercise chosen, the training condition, and the degree of fatigue [188,189]. As a guideline, you can assume that you can perform 30% of your maximum strength (1RM) about 30–60 times, while you can perform 80% of the 1RM 6–12 times. That said, there is significant inter–individual variation, especially with lighter loads, making the task of establishing a definitive repetition recommendation for a given percentage of the 1RM more difficult. Some individuals may have difficulty completing all repetitions, while others may finish well before exhaustion. Therefore, alternative strategies—such as lifting to the point of failure or maintaining some repetitions in reserve—may serve as more effective cues than sticking to a set number of repetitions.

Effort

The prevailing understanding seems to be shifting to the notion that the *intensity of effort* exerted during each set, rather than the load or number of repetitions alone, is the driving factor for muscle hypertrophy. Heavy weights produce high effort after only a few repetitions, while lighter weights require a greater number of repetitions to achieve the similar intensity of effort.

One method of measuring this type of training load is the concept of *time under tension*, which is generally defined as the cumulative duration that a muscle is under a given load. While it is sometimes claimed that a certain time under tension must be reached to stimulate muscle hypertrophy, such a threshold has not yet been scientifically demonstrated.

It is plausible to assume that there is a lower limit below which the intensity of resistance training becomes too low to stimulate strength gains. This threshold is probably around 20% of the 1RM, as indicated by a recent training study [190]. This study showed comparable muscle growth at different exercise intensities. However, an intensity of 20% was not sufficient to stimulate hypertrophy to the same extent as the other training protocols.

What intensity levels are commonly used in gym workouts? A study that examined this very question found that, on average, participants chose a load equivalent to 53% of their 1RM for various exercises [191]. While lifting at this intensity in conjunction with a moderate number of repetitions (e.g., between 5 and 15) can certainly stimulate muscle hypertrophy and improve maximum strength for beginners, such a program is not necessarily optimal, especially for those who already have more training experience.

When it comes to strength gains, the widely accepted belief remains unchanged: Lifting heavy weights produces better results than using lighter weights. Lifting should be performed rapidly and forcefully in the concentric phase to optimize neural adaptations. In a meta–analysis, heavy weights/low reps were compared to light weights/high reps and it was reported that heavier weights (>60% of 1 RM) were associated with greater strength gains compared to lighter weights [192]. However, the differences were not as large as might be expected. Thus, it is possible to increase both muscle mass and strength by using the classic "medium weights," which correspond to about 8–15 repetitions, depending on the muscle group and specific exercise.

There are many different groups of patients and elderly people who cannot or will not exercise with heavy weights. For these people, it is important to know that resistance training with lighter weights can also provide good results. Since several studies have shown that lighter weights can be just as effective as heavier weights in building muscle strength and promoting overall health benefits, this is a viable option for people who cannot perform high–intensity resistance exercise.

In summary, training intensity can be chosen freely if the goal is to increase muscle mass. With lighter weights, it is important to emphasize the total stress on the muscles, approaching failure in each set. To optimize strength gains, relatively heavy weights should be used based on the principle of specificity. However, strength gains can also be expected when lifting lighter weights. Some general recommendations for effective resistance training are summarized in Table 10.1.

Table 10.1.
Summary of key resistance training recommendations depending on training goal.

PRINCIPLE	MAXIMAL STRENGTH	STRENGTH + HYPERTROPHY	EXPLOSIVE STRENGTH AND POWER
Frequency	1–3 t/wk	1–3 t/wk *Training frequency in the higher range can provide a dose–response effect.*	1–3 t/wk
Intensity/ target–RM	1–8 RM	4–20 RM *Approach failure.*	1–10 reps *Intention to do the exercise as rapidly and forcefully as possible.*
Form	Free weights/ machines *Largest training effect in the specific exercise.*	Free weights/machines/ own body *Large muscle groups.*	Free weights/machines/ own body *Largest training effect in the specific exercise.*
Volume	2–12 sets/muscle group/wk *No clear dose–response effect.*	4–15 sets/muscle group/wk *Number of sets in the higher range can provide a dose–response effect.*	2–12 sets/muscle group/wk *Avoid velocity loss.*

SPOTLIGHT
Should you always lift to failure?

. . . .

The short answer to this question is that it may be beneficial to finish a few reps before failure. The stimulatory effect on protein synthesis is probably comparable to that if you lift to failure, but with the advantage of less fatigue. The next set or exercise can then be performed with better quality, and the risk of reducing total training volume due to fatigue decreases. In addition, muscle mass can increase at a similar rate when training close to failure as when training to complete failure [193,194]. Another consideration is that when the set is performed to failure, the speed of the movement in the final repetitions is bound to be low. The magnitude of this loss of velocity during the last repetitions has been shown to be associated with a reduced development of explosive power [195].

Concentric vs. eccentric actions

Eccentric training may be more effective in developing strength and muscle mass than concentric exercise alone, but the differences are quite small [196]. The best strategy seems to be to combine concentric actions with some form of eccentric overload. Eccentric overload can be achieved in a variety of ways, such as assisted spotting or the use of specialized training equipment such as flywheel ergometers.

Overall, exercises that involve some form of eccentric overload appear to be somewhat more effective than training with conventional weights [197]. There may also be differences between concentric and eccentric resistance training in terms of where hypertrophy occurs along the muscle group, i.e., regional differences. Eccentric resistance training results in slightly greater growth in the distal portion of the muscle, whereas concentric training results in greater hypertrophy in the middle portion of the muscles [17].

As mentioned in Chapter 9, the mechanisms of muscle hypertrophy may differ to some extent between concentric and eccentric training. Whereas concentric resistance training appears to lead to an increase in the pennation angle and the addition of sarcomeres arranged in parallel, eccentric training, at least to a greater extent than concentric training, stimulates the addition of sarcomeres in series and thus longer fascicles. This means that eccentric training may be particularly beneficial for speed and power production at long muscle lengths, while concentric training has a positive effect on total force capacity.

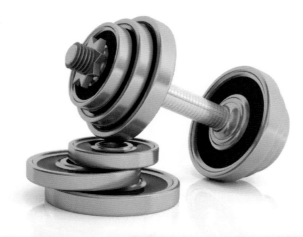

A CLOSER LOOK: Flywheel training

. . . .

In the early 1990s, Swedish researchers Hans Berg and Per Tesch reintroduced resistance training with spinning flywheels. This training method was developed as an exercise program for astronauts to maintain strength and muscle mass in space, since the flywheels are completely independent of gravity. The principle works much like the "yoyo" toy. Conventional weights create a predetermined muscle load that is identical when the weight is lifted and lowered. In contrast, the load in flywheel training is variable and depends on the inertia of the spinning wheel (Fig. 10.1). The trained body part, which is attached to a belt connected to the flywheel, moves back and forth along the desired path. Throughout the concentric phase, the belt is unwound from the flywheel shaft as the rotational speed increases. When the movement is complete, the flywheel continues to rotate and begins to rewind the strap. In this way, eccentric muscle loading is achieved when the rotation of the wheel is slowed by the trainee.

A unique feature of the flywheel is that the stored energy can be freely distributed during the eccentric phase. Without any assistance, the trainee can refrain from braking during the first part of the eccentric action and subsequently achieve a greater eccentric load than was exerted during the concentric phase. It is believed that such eccentric overload is one of the reasons why this form of exercise has proven to be very effective in stimulating muscle hypertrophy and strength in a variety of contexts [197]. Another advantage is that each repetition can, by definition, be performed at the maximum level, since only effort and fatigue set the limit on the force that can be generated.

Figure 10.1.
The principle of flywheel training. During the concentric phase, the person pulls on the belt connected to the shaft of the flywheel. The force is generated by the inertia of the rotating flywheel. When the belt is fully wound, the wheel continues to rotate, but the exerciser must now stop the rotation (eccentric action).

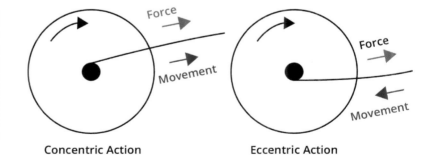

Concentric Action   Eccentric Action

Exercise order

The order of exercises within a session can affect the quality of execution and, ultimately, the muscular adaptations. A rule of thumb is that performance is best at the beginning of a training session. When excessive fatigue is avoided, heavier weights can be lifted, and more repetitions can be performed at a given load. Accordingly, research has shown that strength development is better for exercises scheduled early in the session [198]. Therefore, practical advice is to place priority exercises early in the session.

If the primary goal is muscle hypertrophy, the order of exercise may not matter as much. However, there is evidence that when fatigue sets in, there is a tendency to lift a lower total volume than if the exercise was set at the beginning of the session. A general piece of advice, therefore, is to start with large multi-joint exercises that require attention and coordination, and finish with isolated single-joint exercises and/or supplemental exercises such as core stability.

PERIODIZATION

Periodization is the planned and structured manipulation of various training variables such as intensity, rest time, frequency, and exercise selection within different phases of a training program. The purpose of periodization may be to maximize muscular adaptations, prevent injury, add variety to training, and make it more enjoyable, or to streamline training prior to a specific competition (tapering).

Three main models of periodization are often discussed: linear periodization, undulating periodization, and block periodization. Linear periodization means that training volume is reduced over the course of a given training period while intensity is maintained or increased. With undulating periodization, the volume and intensity vary up and down during the training period. This is usually done on either a weekly or daily basis.

Block periodization comes from competitive sports, where the goal is to perform at the best possible level once or a few times a year. Training is then periodized in different cycles to achieve maximum performance at a given time. Classic blocks within resistance training are strength endurance, hypertrophy, maximum strength, and finally explosiveness or speed and power training.

The question to ask is whether periodization leads to better muscle adaptations than traditional training, which mainly considers the principle of progressive overload. There are several studies in this area and meta-analyzes that have compiled data. Four main conclusions can be drawn from these studies [199]:

- ⮑ Periodized training leads to slightly greater strength improvements than non-periodized training, regardless of training status at the beginning of the training period.
- ⮑ The undulating periodization model leads to slightly better strength improvements than linear periodization, at least in trained individuals.
- ⮑ The importance of periodization can vary between different exercises. For example, periodization has a greater impact on strength development in the bench press than in squats.
- ⮑ Periodization is not important for the development of muscle hypertrophy.

The effect sizes indicate that the boost in strength improvement by periodization is not particularly large, but could still be important in a competitive context. All in all, it appears that proper organization of basic training variables, such as exercise selection, volume, intensity, and the use of progressive overload, is more important than periodization per se.

TIME OF DAY

Is there a specific time of day that most effectively stimulates muscle adaptation to resistance training? One theory is that training should be scheduled based on daily fluctuations in testosterone and/or cortisol levels. These hormones naturally peak in the morning. However, as mentioned earlier in this book, it is doubtful that the natural fluctuations in systemic hormones or the hormonal response to resistance training, in general, have any effect on muscle growth or strength development. There is also no scientific support for the proposition that muscle hypertrophy is optimally stimulated when testosterone levels peak.

Another aspect that has been highlighted is that performance in terms of coordination, reaction time, and muscle strength is generally better in the afternoon when body temperature is higher [200]. Strength levels are usually 5–10% lower in the morning, which is referred to as the ***morning neuromuscular deficit***. It is possible to reduce this deficit by accustoming the body to morning training sessions [201]. Nevertheless, it can be argued that training in the afternoon or evening can lead to better results due to the better quality of training.

In the studies that have compared training in the morning with training in the evening, there are no clear trends in favor of one time of day or the other. A Finnish study found similar muscle hypertrophy regardless of the time of day during a 10–week training program [202]. Similar results were recently obtained in a study that examined both muscle volume and strength in untrained men who were randomly assigned to train either in the morning or in the afternoon for 11 weeks [203].

In summary, time of day does not appear to play a critical role with respect to muscle adaptations to resistance training. Practical aspects and personal preferences can therefore guide the training schedule in this respect.

SPOTLIGHT
Training to optimize muscle hypertrophy
. . . .

This chapter has made it clear that certain training variables are of greater importance than others in optimizing adaptations to resistance training. To optimize muscle hypertrophy, a relatively large volume of exercise should be performed, at least 10 sets per muscle group per week, preferably divided into at least 2 training sessions per week. A combination of multi–joint exercises and isolated exercises can be used, mainly because it is difficult to optimally stimulate all muscle groups in multi–joint exercises. Both concentric and eccentric actions should be included in the training program, including exercises at longer muscle lengths.

Rest time between sets is of little importance as long as fatigue does not result in performing a lower volume of exercise. Therefore, 2–3 minutes of rest between sets may be a suitable guideline. As for the intensity and the number of repetitions per set, you have great freedom as long as the muscles being trained are properly stressed. If you use lighter weights, it is important to approach failure to activate all muscle fibers during the set. Finally, it seems that an internal focus on the muscles being used during the lift gives slightly better results than an external focus [204].

DIFFERENT TYPES OF EXERCISE

Exercise selection

Resistance training offers a variety of options, including bodyweight exercises, machines, free weights, kettlebells, elastic bands, and variable resistance equipment, to name a few. In addition, specialized methods such as plyometric, ballistic, and eccentric training each bring unique aspects to the overall routine. Exercises can target single or multiple joints and be performed unilaterally or bilaterally. While not every resistance training method and exercise is discussed in this book, it is worth noting that each can vary in its ability to stimulate muscle hypertrophy, maximize strength, or improve explosive power.

There are many examples of exercises that target the same muscle group but differ significantly in the degree of muscle activation. For example, in the book Muscle Meets Magnet by Per Tesch, which evaluated numerous exercises using functional magnetic resonance imaging, it was shown that the seated leg curl results in significantly less muscle activation of the hamstring muscles than the stiff–legged deadlift [205]. Those engaged in resistance training should preferably have a basic understanding of the joints and muscle groups targeted by specific exercises, as well as the primary adaptations targeted by those exercises. However, without objective tools, it can be difficult to assess the effectiveness of exercises. Exercises that appear similar at first glance may produce very different results in terms of muscle activation and adaptation.

For optimal results when resistance training in an athletic setting or rehabilitating from an injury, it is important to incorporate a variety of exercises based on a needs assessment. Exercises should be chosen wisely based on the targeted muscle groups, range of motion, speed, loading patterns, and specific requirements of the sport (see Chapter 17).

For recreational athletes who simply want to build muscle and benefit from the overall health effects of resistance training, exercise selection should not be overemphasized. There are numerous approaches to effective resistance training, and a variety of exercises and equipment are available. Ultimately, personal preference is important, and intensity of effort plays a decisive role in the gains achieved.

SPOTLIGHT
Should you exercise with free weights or on machines?

Exercise modality can significantly influence factors such as range of motion, muscle activation, speed of movement, synergist engagement, and overall coordination involvement. This in turn affects the muscular response and adaptation to training. The use of machines is usually safe and user–friendly, but often requires access to a gym. On the other hand, free weights are often touted as superior due to their coordination and balance requirements and purported greater "functional" benefits.

A recent 8–week study comparing these two training methods concluded that both are equally effective in promoting strength and muscle growth without overloading joints [206]. Since there is no one–size–fits–all formula, many people could achieve optimal benefits by combining different training modalities and equipment to promote muscle development and enjoy the benefits of resistance training.

Occlusion training

Restricting blood supply to muscles during resistance training has been shown to be an effective method of rapidly increasing strength and muscle mass despite training with lighter weights. This method is called occlusion training or ischemic resistance training. Typically, a cuff is used to apply pressure that restricts blood flow to the muscle. The main advantage of occlusion training is that it can be done by people who, for some reason, cannot or do not want to train with heavier weights, for example, during rehabilitation after an injury. Typically, a load of about 20–30% of 1RM is used.

The main mechanism why occlusion training works seems to be that fatigue/failure is reached earlier, i.e., after fewer repetitions than when training with comparable weights without restricting blood flow [207,208]. Occlusion training leads to cell swelling, accumulation of metabolites, activation of satellite cells, and marked stimulation of protein synthesis, which explains its effectiveness in promoting hypertrophy. However, there is no strong evidence that occlusion training is better than traditional resistance training (performed close to failure) in stimulating muscle hypertrophy. Despite the relatively low loads, occlusion training also results in significant strength increases.

One disadvantage of occlusion training is that it can be somewhat painful. Following the principle of specificity, it is also difficult to maximize improvement in maximal strength with occlusion training. Nonetheless, strength-oriented individuals can use occlusion training as a possible supplement to their more traditional lifting routines.

Vibration training

Various forms of vibration training have been around for quite some time and are often used in combination with traditional resistance training. Vibration training is touted as effective for increasing muscle activation and developing strength and explosiveness.

In the most common method, vibrations are delivered indirectly to the muscles via vibrating platforms. This is referred to as whole-body vibration training. The vibrations can be adjusted for both amplitude and frequency, and the workout can be either static or dynamic. There are two main types of platforms, with vertical platforms vibrating in the vertical direction, while oscillating platforms rotate in the horizontal plane.

Meta-analyzes have shown that vibration training can help increase strength and power but the effects are not greater than traditional resistance training and results vary greatly depending on the type of vibration platform used, the exercises performed, and the specific vibration protocol [209,210]. Therefore, vibration training, like the occlusion training described above, should be considered as a complement rather than a replacement for other forms of resistance training.

SPOTLIGHT
Training to optimize explosiveness
. . . .

The ability to develop as much force as possible as quickly as possible is called "explosiveness". The goal of these powerful actions is to generate maximum speed and power during various lifts, jumps, brakes, or changes of direction. Maximum force and power are fundamentally linked, as stronger individuals usually develop greater peak power. Therefore, almost all forms of resistance training that increase maximum strength also increase explosiveness. For well-trained individuals, a combination of heavy resistance training and more specific explosive exercises is likely required to improve this ability. Therefore, to develop explosiveness, a combination of exercises is often used that includes traditional heavy resistance training, ballistic exercises, weightlifting exercises, and various jumps. The exercises should always be performed as explosively as possible.

The advantage of traditional resistance training with normal weights is that a high load is possible, but unfortunately the braking/deceleration portion of the exercises is significant. Ballistic training (in which an object, such as a medicine ball, is accelerated throughout the movement and then released) can therefore be used to eliminate the deceleration phase and allow for high speed and power development.

In plyometric exercises, the stretch-shortening cycle is used to quickly switch between the eccentric and concentric phases during different jumps. This type of training should preferably be performed with high specificity for the action to be improved (e.g., a sport-specific action). Weightlifting exercises such as the clean and jerk can be used as an additional supplement, as these exercises are associated with high power development, albeit for a limited number of movements.

Explosive training stimulates the activation of the nervous system and the contractility of the muscles. Adaptations in the tendon and connective tissue are also important, as increased stiffness in these complexes is associated with improved force transfer from muscle to bone, and thus an increased rate of force development. Finally, it should be noted that many explosive exercises, not least plyometric jumps, are stressful to muscles, tendons and connective tissue, and therefore require adequate recovery between training sessions.

SUMMARY

- ⮑ The basic training principles for resistance training include the principles of overload, specificity, and reversibility.

- ⮑ Exercise variables that are important to training outcomes include intensity (load), frequency, volume, and intensity of effort.

- ⮑ There is a clear dose-response relationship between exercise volume and muscle hypertrophy, with muscle growth benefiting from higher volume, at least up to 10 sets per muscle group per week.

- ⮑ Training frequency is relevant because higher training frequency usually leads to greater total training volume. In volume-based comparisons of different training frequencies, training frequency does not seem to play a decisive role.

- The length of rest between sets and exercises may affect short-term performance in the next set or exercise, but also longer-term adaptations.

- To optimize muscular adaptations, relatively long rests are recommended (2–5 minutes). However, short rests boost the cardiovascular system and save time.

- Exercise intensity or load is not critical to the hypertrophic response. Muscle growth can be stimulated with both heavier and lighter loads. However, with lighter loads, it becomes more important to approach failure with each set.

- To optimize strength gains, the principle of specificity dictates that relatively heavy loads should be used. However, significant strength gains can also be expected with lighter loads.

- Eccentric training may be more effective in developing strength and muscle mass compared to purely concentric exercises, but the differences are quite small. Therefore, it is recommended to combine concentric and eccentric exercises to optimize adaptations to resistance training.

- The order of exercises during a session can be relevant to consider, as performance is best in the rested/non-fatigued state. Therefore, a practical recommendation is to perform the most important and technically demanding exercises early in the session.

- Periodization means varying training variables such as intensity, rest time, frequency, and exercise selection in a planned and structured manner within different phases (cycles) of a training program.

- Periodization is not important for muscle hypertrophy. Progressive overload and a high total training volume are sufficient to maximize muscle growth.

- Periodized training may result in slightly greater strength improvements than non-periodized training, regardless of training status at the start of the training program.

- Performance is generally better in the afternoon and evening than in the morning. Nevertheless, research studies have found no differences in training effects between morning and afternoon training. Personal preferences may therefore guide the scheduling of training sessions.

- There are a number of different resistance training methods and exercises to choose from, and the choice of exercise and equipment can be important to the adaptive response.

- Restricting blood flow to muscles during resistance training (occlusion training) has been shown to be an effective method for rapidly increasing strength and muscle mass despite training with lighter loads. However, there is no strong evidence that occlusion training per se is better than conventional resistance training in stimulating muscle hypertrophy or strength.

- Vibration training can be used as a complement to traditional resistance training to develop muscle strength and power.

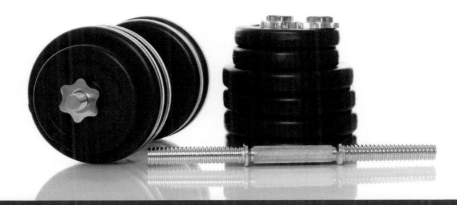

CHAPTER 11

THE ROLE OF PROTEIN INTAKE

The relationship between protein consumption and resistance exercise is a widely discussed topic in fitness and sports. Our skeletal muscle tissue is not only a fluid reservoir, but also consists largely of proteins, which make up about 20% of its wet weight. This abundance of proteins in muscle is in constant flux and is subject to a cycle of synthesis and degradation, with about 1–2% of the total protein pool being recycled daily (see Chapter 4). In general, this process maintains equilibrium throughout the day, with protein synthesis and degradation occurring at approximately equal rates. This results in a stable net protein balance, with an equal amount of muscle tissue being built and broken down. However, this balance can be disrupted by resistance training, a strong anabolic stimulus. Resistance training primarily increases protein synthesis, which, in conjunction with dietary proteins, can lead to a progressive increase in muscle mass over time. In this chapter, we take a closer look at the importance of protein intake in facilitating muscular adaptations in response to resistance training.

PROTEIN NEEDS

A prerequisite for assuming that resistance training is an anabolic stimulus is that we consume protein at some point during the day. Amino acids, which come from proteins ingested with food, are the building blocks of protein synthesis. There are 9 essential amino acids that the body cannot produce itself and that have already been mentioned in Chapter 2. Many of the proteins that occur naturally in food, for example in meat, chicken, fish, eggs, and milk, are so-called high-quality proteins and contain all the essential amino acids.

The fact that the body needs protein to build muscle mass does not necessarily mean that it is difficult to meet the basic protein requirement, which for the total population is given as 0.8 g of protein per kg of body weight per day. On the contrary, questionnaires show that most people meet their basic protein needs through the diet, even those who exercise regularly. There is a correlation between total energy intake and protein intake. For example, people with high energy expenditure (due to a high body mass and/or a high level of physical activity) naturally consume more protein. Most people who eat a reasonably mixed diet can therefore meet their daily protein requirements with normal foods.

However, individuals who engage in resistance training require a higher protein intake than their inactive counterparts. While the recommended daily protein intake for the general population is 0.8 g/kg/day, based primarily on nitrogen balance measurements, a more reasonable target for resistance training participants is approximately 1.6 g/kg/day [211], a topic to which we will return.

OPTIMIZATION OF PROTEIN SYNTHESIS DURING RESISTANCE TRAINING

Protein intake has a major impact on protein synthesis after exercise. When protein is consumed, the net protein balance becomes positive and the anabolic effects of resistance training can take effect. This has led many people to believe that the timing of protein intake relative to the training session is critical to the subsequent adaptive response in skeletal muscles. We will return to this question after examining the factors that influence protein synthesis in the context of resistance training.

Protein quantity

An intake of about 20 grams of protein provides near-maximal stimulation of protein synthesis after resistance training [212]. If a whole-body exercise program is performed, 40 grams may have a slightly greater effect than 20 grams [213], but whether this matters for the long-term training response is uncertain.

Pooling data from several studies, it appears that 0.25 g/kg/day optimizes the protein synthetic response in young, healthy individuals. However, in older people, this value can be as high as 0.40 g/kg/day [214], suggesting that older people need to consume more protein relative to body weight than younger people to optimize muscular protein balance. The anabolic response to resistance training and amino acid consumption is therefore attenuated in the elderly, which is referred to as **anabolic resistance.** This is one of the reasons why it might be advisable for older people to review their daily protein intake.

Protein quality

Different protein sources may differ in how effectively they can stimulate protein synthesis. Efficiency is determined by how quickly the protein is broken down and absorbed, as well as the specific amino acid profile. Whey protein stimulates protein synthesis better than casein because whey contains a greater amount of essential amino acids, including leucine [215]. Animal proteins contain a large amount of essential amino acids and are therefore generally more effective than plant proteins in stimulating protein synthesis [216]. Milk protein, for example, stimulates protein synthesis better than soy protein [217]. However, possible deficiencies of a plant–based diet in terms of protein quality can be adequately compensated for by simply increasing protein intake from various plant sources to ensure that all amino acids are consumed in sufficient quantity. Furthermore, there is currently no evidence of a significant difference between plant–based and omnivorous diets in terms of muscle growth after exercise.

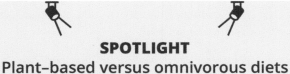

SPOTLIGHT
Plant–based versus omnivorous diets

· · · · · · · · · · · · · · · · · · · ·

In one notable study, researchers found that muscle strength and hypertrophy were equally enhanced by two different types of high–protein diets: a plant-only diet consisting of whole plant foods supplemented with soy protein isolate, and a mixed diet containing a variety of whole foods supplemented with whey protein [218]. This strongly suggests that the specific protein source— whether plant or animal—does not significantly influence the muscle adaptations elicited by resistance training. Instead, the key determinant of effective muscle building and strength gains appears to be the ingestion of an adequate amount of protein, regardless of whether it is derived from plant or animal sources.

The amino acid that is most effective in stimulating protein synthesis is leucine. However, the other amino acids are also important, and there is no additional effect of leucine if the protein of a particular meal already contains enough essential amino acids. However, if protein intake is low, supplementation of leucine or branched–chain amino acids can have a stimulating effect on protein synthesis. Nevertheless, building new muscle proteins ultimately requires the involvement of all amino acids, underscoring their collective importance in muscle growth and repair.

Simultaneous intake of other macronutrients

Because of the insulin–secreting properties of carbohydrates, it has been postulated that their consumption prior to exercise could promote protein synthesis and reduce protein breakdown. However, research to date indicates that concurrent carbohydrate intake does not result in improved muscle protein balance when protein intake is adjusted to recommended levels [219]. In fact, normal insulin concentrations have a minimal effect on protein synthesis [144], and the amounts of insulin required to inhibit protein breakdown are similarly small. Furthermore, supplementing a protein bolus with fat does not appear to affect protein synthesis rates [220].

THE IMPORTANCE OF PROTEIN TIMING

Protein supplementation enhances the protein synthetic response to resistance training, resulting in a favorable net muscle protein balance. Contrary to the notion that protein must be ingested immediately after training, resistance training itself serves as the key anabolic stimulus. The trained muscle continues to respond to protein intake for up to 24 hours after exercise [221]. This observation refutes the idea of a single "window" for protein intake, although it may be more practical to spread protein intake over several meals. The overarching conclusion is that total daily protein intake is more important than timing of intake. Accordingly, protein intake before or after exercise could promote muscle mass adaptation if it contributes to increased total daily protein intake to the desired target level.

In the most comprehensive meta–analysis examining protein intake in the context of chronic resistance training, the main findings were [211]:

- ➲ Protein supplementation significantly enhanced the effects of resistance training on strength and muscle mass, with the effects being most pronounced in already trained individuals.

- ➲ The positive effect on muscle mass decreased with age, and no further benefits were observed when protein intake exceeded 1.6 g/kg/day (Fig. 11.1).

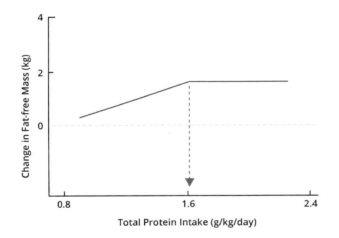

Figure 11.1.
Changes in lean body mass with different protein intakes. The figure shows that a protein intake of about 1.6 g/kg/day produces near maximum effect, although with considerable variance. Based on data from Morton et al. 2018. The complete reference can be found in the Figure references section at the end of the book.

Based on current scientific evidence, the recommended protein intake is between 20–40 grams per meal, distributed over 4–5 meals daily. Consuming a high–protein snack or supplement near the time of exercise may be beneficial if it contributes to a higher total daily protein intake. For individuals already consuming more than 1.6 g/kg/day, the timing of protein intake is less critical; a short period of fasting after exercise is unlikely to be detrimental when preparing a subsequent meal.

Protein supplements are a convenient means of achieving daily protein goals to optimize the effects of resistance training. They are also relatively inexpensive compared to some whole foods. For example, the cost per gram of protein is higher for milk than for a whey protein shake. However, whole foods are equally effective at stimulating muscle protein synthesis, although direct comparisons in the scientific literature are sparse. Low–quality protein sources, such as some plant proteins, can be compensated for by a slight increase in total intake.

In summary, the main goal for individuals engaged in resistance training should be a balanced diet that not only meets adequate protein requirements, but also contains important macro– and micronutrients [222].

PROTEIN CONSUMPTION PRIOR TO SLEEP

Numerous studies have examined the effects of protein intake before bedtime on protein synthesis at night. While this strategy has been shown to increase protein synthesis during the night, no study to date has demonstrated its superiority compared with protein intake at other times of the day. The main benefit of protein intake before bedtime appears to be an increase in total daily protein intake [223]. This is especially important for the elderly, who often eat fewer meals and less protein–rich foods. Therefore, protein intake before bedtime proves to be a practical way to increase protein intake and increase muscle protein turnover overnight without compromising appetite for breakfast the next morning [224].

SPOTLIGHT
Can a high protein intake be harmful?
. . . .

There is a plethora of beliefs, some of which are even promoted in textbooks, that a high–protein diet can have detrimental effects on the kidneys or skeletal structures. However, a thorough examination of the research literature provides no evidence to support such claims in the context of healthy individuals. These misconceptions come primarily from studies conducted in patients with existing kidney dysfunction. In individuals without health complications, a daily protein intake of about 3 g/kg/day over an extended period of time appears to be safe [225-227]. Nevertheless, it is important to note that the long–term health effects of a very high protein diet are not yet well defined. Even if a high–protein diet does not directly lead to health problems, it may have drawbacks, such as neglecting other vital nutrients or risking excessive calorie consumption that could gradually lead to an increase in fat mass. Overall, there seems to be little reason to go much beyond the recommended dose of about 1.6 g/kg/day for optimal response to resistance training.

SUMMARY

- ⊃ A prerequisite for the anabolic effect of resistance training is the intake of protein at some point during the day.

- ⊃ The recommended daily protein intake for the general population is about 0.8 g/kg/day. The vast majority of people who eat a reasonably mixed diet meet the basic protein requirements with normal food.

- ⊃ The optimal daily intake for people engaged in resistance training appears to be about 1.6 g/kg/day.

- ⊃ Intakes of complete proteins, essential amino acids, or branched–chain amino acids stimulate muscle protein synthesis in conjunction with resistance training.

- ⊃ An intake equivalent to 0.25 g/kg/day optimizes the protein synthesis response in young healthy individuals. In older people, this value is 0.40 g/kg/day, which means that it can be more difficult for older people to optimize muscle protein balance.

- ⊃ Leucine is the single amino acid that most effectively stimulates protein synthesis, but all amino acids are needed for building muscle mass.

- ⊃ Possible shortcomings of a plant–based diet in terms of protein quality can be adequately compensated by simply increasing the total protein intake and varying the sources.

- ⊃ When the recommended amount of protein is consumed, the simultaneous intake of carbohydrates or fats has no additional effect on protein balance.

- ⊃ To optimize protein balance in the short term and muscle mass in the long term, total daily protein intake is more important than the timing of intake.

- ⊃ Protein supplementation has a small, but still positive effect on muscle mass and strength when combined with resistance training.

- ⊃ The effect of protein supplementation is greater in trained individuals than in untrained individuals, and in younger compared to older individuals.

- ⊃ Taking protein before bed may have a positive effect on muscle protein balance during the night, but any positive effects on muscle mass are primarily due to an increase in total protein intake.

- ⊃ There is no scientific evidence that high protein intake is harmful for healthy people, but there may still be disadvantages with very high intakes.

CHAPTER 12

DIETARY SUPPLEMENTS FOR RESISTANCE TRAINING

The dietary supplement industry is a huge business, fueled mainly by the search for convenient and quick solutions to improve results in the gym or promote health. More than half of all gym-goers regularly incorporate some form of nutritional supplements into their routine. But which of these supplements are useful for resistance training? Before we explore this question, we will first define what a dietary supplement is.

DEFINITION OF DIETARY SUPPLEMENTS

There are several different definitions of dietary supplements. The International Olympic Committee definition is as follows [228]:

> "A food, food component, nutrient, or non–food compound that is purposefully introduced in addition to the habitually consumed diet with the aim of achieving a specific health and/or performance benefit."

Thus, dietary supplements are intentionally taken over and above the normal diet with the specific goal of improving health or performance parameters. In the general population, vitamins, minerals, antioxidants, or essential fatty acids are often supplemented in hopes of improving health or correcting nutritional deficiencies.

Athletes often consume macronutrients in more concentrated forms, such as high–carbohydrate gels, bars, and sports drinks, or high–protein shakes and bars. In addition to supplements that meet additional carbohydrate and protein needs, supplements such as caffeine and creatine are common among people engaged in resistance training. These types of supplements are usually grouped under **ergogenic supplements** as they are believed to have a performance–enhancing effect.

WHY USE SUPPLEMENTS?

Why do elite and recreational athletes use nutritional supplements? The following reasons have been highlighted [228]:

- ➲ To correct or prevent a deficiency in a particular nutrient, such as vitamins or minerals
- ➲ To provide an easy, quick, and efficient supply of energy and nutrients during exercise
- ➲ To achieve a specific performance enhancement before a competition or game
- ➲ To achieve an indirect increase in performance by allowing you to train harder, recover faster, or reduce the risk of injury and a weakened immune system
- ➲ For financial reasons, such as sponsorship or to receive free products from a company
- ➲ As an insurance policy, on a "just in case" basis.
- ➲ Because other athletes on the same team or in the same sport use nutritional supplements

Many people use supplements unnecessarily. For health purposes, various supplements are used to support the immune system, e.g., various vitamins, minerals, and antioxidants. For people who eat a mixed diet, these supplements are usually unnecessary. However, when deficiencies have been identified, some micronutrients can have a positive effect. This is especially true of vitamin D, iron, and calcium. In this book, however, the focus is on supplements that may affect the outcome of resistance training.

WHICH DIETARY SUPPLEMENTS WORK?

There is an abundance of different dietary supplements. The most popular supplements relevant to resistance training are listed in Table 12.1. Some established supplements that are almost exclusively associated with endurance or sprint exercise, such as sports drinks (carbohydrate solutions), nitrates, and bicarbonate, are not listed here.

Table 12.1.
Summary of the most established dietary supplements relevant to resistance training.

SUPPLEMENT	PROPOSED MECHANISM OF ACTION	EVIDENCE
Protein supplement	Provides the body with amino acids to build muscle tissue. Increases protein synthesis in conjunction with resistance training.	Strong evidence of a positive (but small) effect, especially when supplementation results in increased intake up to a dose of about 1.6 g/kg/day.
Caffeine	Adenosine receptor antagonism, increased release of endorphins, improved neuromuscular performance, increased alertness, and decreased fatigue.	Strong evidence of beneficial effects during supramaximal sprints, intermittent work, and prolonged endurance work. Emerging evidence of a small effect on strength–related outcome measures.
Beta–alanine	Increases intracellular buffering capacity.	Small but potentially important effects on endurance performance and repeated sprints, unclear and relatively unexplored effects related to resistance training.
Creatine	Increased creatine phosphate and intracellular fluid, improved recovery, and increased expression of growth factors.	Strong evidence of improved development of strength and muscle mass associated with resistance training, as well as enhanced performance during repetitive high–intensity work.
Omega–3	Possibly increased protein synthesis, anti–inflammatory effects leading to reduced symptoms of exercise–induced muscle soreness and accelerated recovery of muscle function.	Some evidence of accelerated recovery after eccentric work and increased muscle mass in the elderly, but generally conflicting data.
HMB	Increased protein synthesis and decreased protein breakdown, increased activation of satellite cells.	Although individual studies have indicated positive effects, the general view is that HMB has no ergogenic effect when protein intake is already optimal.

The table shows that several dietary supplements have moderate to strong empirical support for affecting certain performance variables. However, when looking at the parameters related to resistance training — namely muscle mass, strength, exercise capacity, and recovery — only a limited number of supplements show ergogenic effects. Protein supplements and creatine receive strong support, while caffeine and omega–3 fatty acids receive only moderate support. It is worth noting that adequate protein intake can be achieved through a balanced diet, so supplementation is not essential (but may be practical). Creatine thus stands out as the supplement with strong empirical support that is difficult to obtain in effective doses through diet alone.

The typical protocol for creatine supplementation includes a loading phase of 20 grams per day (divided into four different doses) for 5–7 days, followed by a maintenance phase of 3–5 grams per day. However, creatine is not a magic muscle–building supplement — proper resistance training is required and the effects achieved can vary from individual to individual. Nevertheless, most people can expect small but positive effects from creatine supplementation [229].

RISKS AND DISADVANTAGES OF DIETARY SUPPLEMENTS

There are several risks and disadvantages to dietary supplements. This is also the reason why many sports organizations recommend dietary supplements only restrictively. The less serious disadvantages are that supplements are generally expensive and unnecessary for most people. The more serious risks are that some supplements may have a direct negative impact on health. There is no guarantee that the content claimed on the packaging will match the actual contents of the product. There is also a small risk of accidental doping through contaminated products or products that are mistaken for banned substances such as anabolic steroids, even if this is not indicated in the list of ingredients.

When the doping laboratory in Cologne examined over 600 dietary supplements purchased over the Internet, it was found that 15% of them contained banned substances that would have resulted in a positive doping test [230]. Even a very small amount of a banned molecule in a product is enough to cause a positive test. Some dietary supplements have also been found to contain higher levels of endocrine disruptors than can be considered acceptable [231].

Minimizing the risk

The most important step in reducing the risks associated with dietary supplements is to become informed about their potential benefits and risks. This knowledge should help us avoid supplements that have little or no effect or that are associated with risks that exceed acceptable levels. In general, products that boast bold claims and exaggerated promises on their labels should be approached with caution and skepticism. For example, there is no dietary supplement that can significantly increase fat burning and weight loss.

It is advisable to purchase dietary supplements from reputable companies. Products from trusted pharmacies carry fewer risks than those from obscure websites that make lofty claims. A careful review of the ingredients list can ensure that the product does not contain substances that are classified as doping agents. Athletes should ideally seek advice from professionals at their sports club or gym.

Even though some supplements have small positive effects, the focus should be on obtaining clean, effective products through the safest possible channels. It is important to remember that dietary supplements cannot replace a balanced, healthy diet. The "food first approach" is a commonly held principle.

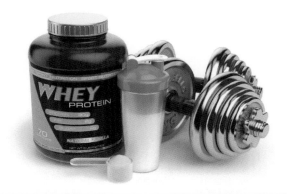

SUMMARY

⮁ A dietary supplement is a food or dietary ingredient taken over and above the normal diet for the purpose of improving a specific health or performance parameter.

⮁ There are many different reasons why individuals engaged in resistance training take nutritional supplements.

⮁ When specific deficiencies have been identified, supplementing with various micronutrients such as iron, calcium, or vitamin D can have a positive effect.

⮁ Among supplements reported to influence muscle mass or strength in conjunction with resistance training, there is strong evidence for the beneficial effects of protein supplements and creatine, and moderate/emerging evidence for caffeine and omega–3 fatty acids.

⮁ There are several potential risks and drawbacks to dietary supplements, not the least of which are cost, risk of overdose, and risk of contamination or misrepresented ingredients and thus misuse and/or adverse effects.

⮁ Dietary supplements should not replace a healthy and balanced diet according to the "food first approach" principle.

CHAPTER 13

MUSCLE FATIGUE AND EXERCISE-INDUCED MUSCLE DAMAGE

Most people have probably experienced the feeling of muscle fatigue and muscle damage after exercise at some point in their lives. Muscle fatigue, the immediate result of strenuous exercise, manifests itself as a temporary reduction in the muscle's ability to perform optimally. In contrast, muscle damage after exercise — also referred to as "delayed onset muscle soreness" or DOMS — usually becomes noticeable in the days following exercise and causes discomfort and stiffness. This chapter addresses the underlying physiological mechanisms responsible for muscle fatigue and exercise-induced muscle damage.

MUSCLE FATIGUE

Muscle fatigue can be described as the diminishing of muscle strength even though maximum effort is exerted during a contraction. A fatigued muscle is both weaker and slower than a non–fatigued muscle, both in terms of shortening and relaxation. In addition, the precision of the intended movements is impaired. Muscle function recovers relatively quickly after rest, from a few seconds to several hours, depending on the circumstances. In some cases, residual strength loss may last several days due to exercise–induced muscle damage.

It is difficult to rely solely on human studies when attempting to elucidate the mechanisms of muscle fatigue. Relevant findings have been obtained from a combination of human studies, animal studies, and isolated experiments on individual muscle fibers. While the causes of muscle fatigue may vary depending on the type and intensity of exercise, they are often classified as central or peripheral in origin. Central fatigue includes all aspects of motor control that involve the central nervous system, i.e., all the way from the brain to the axon terminal. Peripheral fatigue includes all processes from the motor endplate to the cross–bridge cycle of myofibrils. Central and peripheral mechanisms of fatigue can occur simultaneously and influence each other. In addition to training mode, intensity, and duration, fatigue is also influenced by overall fitness and training status, as well as external factors such as the environment (e.g., temperature and altitude).

The following is a brief overview of the most common mechanisms proposed to cause, or at least contribute to, muscle fatigue during resistance training. The etiology of muscle fatigue in more traditional endurance competitions or team sports may differ to some degree from the following summary.

Central fatigue

It is difficult to activate muscles to the absolute maximum. However, when lifting loads that require maximum effort, most available motor units, including the largest and fastest, are recruited. There is a central part of muscle fatigue that involves the readiness and alertness of the central nervous system, which is called "arousal." Evidence that arousal can affect muscle strength comes from studies in which subjects received strong verbal encouragement or other stimulation while lifting heavy loads. Recruitment of motor units then increases slightly, and so does maximum force. This supports the hypothesis that central factors may limit force production. Indeed, some studies have reported a reduced ability to maximally activate muscles during fatiguing resistance training [184,232].

The role of the brain in central fatigue has been controversial for decades. One widely cited theory is that the brain acts as a "***central governor***," controlling the level of fiber activation based on the various inputs the brain receives during physical work. Perhaps the most compelling evidence for the brain's role in fatigue comes from pharmacological interventions that have found that various central stimulants (such as amphetamine) can enhance performance [233]. The importance of the brain in fatigue has also been recognized in recent years, as several studies have shown positive effects on performance from carbohydrate mouth–rinsing. Since performance is improved even though the carbohydrates are not absorbed by the gut, it is believed that the sugar acts on the brain in some way so that performance increases [234].

The relative importance of the central versus peripheral nervous system in muscle fatigue probably depends on the type of exercise performed. However, most researchers seem to agree that peripheral fatigue factors that directly affect contractile function are of greater importance than central fatigue during resistance training.

Lactic acid/lactate

An accumulation of lactate in muscles has long been cited as a cause of muscle fatigue. Even people outside of sports have heard of lactate and are aware of its connection to fatigue. When people talk about lactic acid, they usually mean lactate and the hydrogen ions associated with lactate formation. Lactate is formed during the anaerobic breakdown of muscle glycogen. An increased amount of hydrogen ions results in a lowered pH in muscle, and there are many types of experiments showing that a lowered pH can affect the function of many different tissues.

Nevertheless, research suggests that lactate and low pH are not the primary causes of peripheral muscle fatigue. Skeletal muscle is less sensitive to low pH than many other cell types. Lowering muscle pH to a level that occurs with fatigue does not reduce muscle function [235]. Nor is there direct evidence that lactate or lowered pH contribute to central fatigue.

The reason lactate is linked with fatigue is probably the notion that rising blood lactate levels often coincides with fatigue. This is simply because intense work depends largely on anaerobic processes to produce ATP, and the anaerobic breakdown of carbohydrates produces large amounts of lactate, which can be measured in the blood during and after intense physical work.

Potassium

Some researchers have suggested that the accumulation of potassium around the muscle membrane may be one of the causes of muscle fatigue [236]. During intense muscle activity, action potentials are fired at a high frequency, resulting in an accumulation of potassium ions outside the muscle cell. This has a negative effect on the sodium–potassium pump. However, when isolated muscles were examined in a solution with increased potassium concentration, fatigue was not exacerbated [237], suggesting that the sodium–potassium pump also functions during muscle fatigue. The significance of increased extracellular potassium levels for muscle fatigue is therefore unclear.

Inorganic phosphates and calcium handling

The breakdown of phosphocreatine is an important source of ATP for intense muscle work. Phosphocreatine is broken down into free creatine and phosphate ions, a reaction facilitated by the enzyme creatine kinase. The increased concentration of phosphate ions has been shown to play an important role in the onset of muscle fatigue. Experimental evidence for this comes mainly from isolated experiments with mice lacking creatine kinase and from experiments in which creatine kinase was injected [238,239]. In particular, the free phosphate ions accumulated by the breakdown of phosphocreatine have been shown to impair the force–producing phase of the cross–bridge cycle in myofibrils. In addition, phosphate accumulation leads to impaired contractile function by interfering with calcium balance in the muscle cell. All in all, the accumulation of phosphate ions seems to be the main cause of impaired calcium release and decreased calcium sensitivity [235]. Together, this leads to weakened cross–bridge function and decreased force production.

Glycogen

Muscle glycogen depletion is closely related to muscle fatigue, not least in endurance sports where glycogen reserves are said to be depleted when you "hit the wall." However, glycogen levels can also play a role in shorter–term work, such as resistance training. Muscles with low glycogen levels fatigue more quickly than muscles with fully loaded glycogen stores [240]. However, the relationship between force production and impaired calcium balance caused by free phosphate ions appears to be the same regardless of high or low glycogen levels. Thus, muscles with low glycogen stores fatigue more quickly because phosphate ion concentrations increase more rapidly. The impaired handling of calcium therefore occurs earlier in intense work with low glycogen content [241].

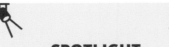

SPOTLIGHT
Why can't you lift your 1RM twice?
. . . .

The question of which fatigue mechanisms contribute most to decreased force production becomes clear when you ask yourself the simple question of why you can't lift your 1RM twice. Research suggests that this is due to an immediate accumulation of phosphate ions that negatively impacts cross-bridge function. This accumulation of phosphate ions also relatively quickly impairs myofibril calcium sensitivity and results in less calcium release from the sarcoplasmic reticulum. Thus, the peripheral causes of muscle fatigue can be divided into three distinct components:

- ⮑   Impaired cross-bridge function due to phosphate ion accumulation
- ⮑   Decreased calcium sensitivity of myofibrils
- ⮑   Decreased calcium release from the sarcoplasmic reticulum

A prerequisite for these factors to limit force production is that neural activation of the muscles has been maximal. If this has not been the case, the decreased force production may also be due to central fatigue.

EXERCISE-INDUCED MUSCLE DAMAGE

In the scientific literature, the delayed sensation of muscle pain after exercise is referred to as **exercise-induced muscle damage** (EIMD) or **delayed-onset muscle soreness** (DOMS). The time course of EIMD can range from almost immediate symptoms to effects that last at least a week after the exercise session. The most common effects of EIMD are impaired muscle function (strength), limited range of motion, and pain/soreness.

The time course and severity of symptoms depend on the type of exercise performed, the individual's training status, and the intensity and duration of training. EIMD is often most severe after exercises that involve eccentric muscle actions. Therefore, resistance training, downhill running, and various sports that involve intermittent, high-intensity work with many changes in direction, such as team sports, are often associated with EIMD.

The typical time course of events associated with EIMD is shown in Figure 13.1. Muscle soreness usually peaks between 24 and 48 hours after exercise and gradually subsides over the following days. The inflammatory processes follow approximately the same time course as the muscle soreness. Impaired muscle function can be 15–50% and is most severe immediately after exercise and then gradually recovers. It can take up to 96 hours for strength to fully return to baseline levels. In very severe EIMD, the impaired function may last even longer. Interestingly, female participants appear less susceptible to EIMD than male participants of the same age [242].

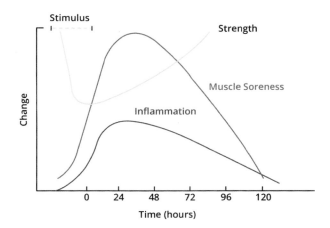

Figure 13.1.
Overview of events associated with exercise-induced muscle damage.

A proven concept related to EIMD is the ***repeated-bout effect***. This means that after an episode of muscle soreness, the muscle is better protected the next time it is subjected to a similar load. Of course, the time between workouts must not be too long for this principle to take effect, but EIMD is likely to be less pronounced even if several weeks have passed between workouts.

The mechanisms behind the repeated bout effect are poorly understood and may include neural, cellular, mechanical, and extracellular matrix adaptations. There is some evidence that longitudinal addition of sarcomeres and adaptations in the inflammatory response occur after the initial eccentric loading, which may help explain the effect [243].

Mechanisms for EIMD

Strong eccentric muscle actions cause small micro damages to the muscle fibers, especially around the Z-discs. In addition, active protein breakdown of structural and contractile proteins occurs. Although the cause of the perceived muscle soreness is not fully understood, it is likely due to an interaction between the structural damage to the muscle fibers causing cell swelling, the invasion of immune cells into the damaged areas, and the disturbed calcium balance in the fibers [244].

The inflammatory response is controlled in part by the enzyme cyclooxygenase, which coordinates the production of prostaglandins. Inflammation is important to cleanse the damaged tissue and initiate the repair and healing processes. There are different types of immune cells that infiltrate the damaged tissue, including neutrophils, mast cells, T lymphocytes and eosinophils.

Some research articles distinguish between the primary and secondary phases of the mechanisms behind EIMD. The primary phase begins with the high mechanical load. Damage to muscle fibers is more pronounced during eccentric muscle actions, in part because eccentric actions are performed with less activation of motor units for a given force compared to concentric or isometric actions. Thus, the greater mechanical stress of eccentric actions is distributed to fewer fibers.

During the moment of mechanical tension, some of the sarcomeres are stretched to the point that they no longer overlap with other myofilaments. The sarcomeres can then "pop" out of position, which has been described as the "***popping sarcomere***" hypothesis [245]. This is an example of the primary structural microinjuries seen in the context of intense exercise leading to EIMD. The primary phase usually includes the impaired contractility observed immediately after the training session. This impaired muscle function is related to muscle fatigue, which was described earlier in the chapter.

In the second phase of EIMD, calcium leakage occurs in the cytoplasm of the muscle. The high calcium levels activate various signaling cascades that increase protein degradation. At very high calcium levels, mitochondria may also be damaged. Elevated calcium levels are also sometimes associated with uncontrolled muscle contractions. This may explain the increased passive tension that often occurs in severe EIMD.

The subsequent inflammatory cascade is a hallmark of the secondary phase of EIMD. The purpose of the inflammatory response is to remove damaged proteins and initiate the repair process. The various immune cells all have specific functions. Neutrophils infiltrate the muscle first, which is driven by the increased calcium content in muscle cells. Neutrophil phagocytes ("eat") degraded tissue and other debris that has formed at the primary lesion. Macrophages (activated monocytes) also play an important role in the inflammatory process and subsequent healing.

Since muscle fibers do not undergo cell division, there is no mechanism to replace damaged fibers. Instead, muscle fibers undergo very extensive repair and remodeling processes so that the fibers eventually function normally again, or preferably even better than before the injury. Satellite cells play an important role in this regeneration process. As mentioned earlier, the satellite cells are the dormant stem cells of the muscles, located between the sarcolemma and the basal lamina. During resistance training, especially during programs involving eccentric actions, these satellite cells are activated and begin to divide.

The exact role of satellite cells in recovery from muscle damage is not yet fully understood, but studies have shown that muscle fiber regeneration is hindered by the absence of satellite cells. Overall, satellite cells have been associated with several different events that are thought to be important in the healing of muscle tissue and, therefore, in recovery after EIMD.

Strategies to reduce EIMD

There are a number of different methods that have been tested to alleviate the symptoms of EIMD or speed recovery, such as stretching and massage. In addition, many different supplements, nutrients, and so-called "functional foods" have been studied. Overall, most of the strategies tested are ineffective.

Protein/amino acid supplementation does not appear to reduce EIMD or speed recovery of muscle function. As for protein, this is quite logical, since muscular protein turnover is about 1–2% per day, whereas the acute muscular stresses associated with EIMD occur quite rapidly and then disappear within a few days. Although activities such as massage, stretching, and compression garments can provide a sense of relief and a perceived reduction in muscle soreness, concrete evidence of their actual effectiveness is still weak.

Dietary polyphenols have been shown to have both antioxidant and anti-inflammatory effects and have therefore been studied for their effect on EIMD. These are abundant in fruits, vegetables, and berries. The most promising results have been obtained in studies on pomegranates and tart cherries [244]. Taken collectively, however, a Cochrane review found that there is limited evidence that antioxidants reduce EIMD [246].

SUMMARY

- ➲ Muscle fatigue can be defined as reduced muscle strength despite maximum voluntary effort to produce the strongest possible contraction.

- ➲ A fatigued muscle is both weaker and slower than a rested muscle, both in terms of shortening and relaxation.

- The causes of muscle fatigue can vary depending on the type and intensity of exercise, but can be independently classified as either "central" or "peripheral" in origin.

- Central fatigue includes all aspects of motor control of muscles by the central nervous system, i.e., all the way from the brain to the axon terminal at the motor end plate.

- Peripheral fatigue includes all processes from the motor end plate to the cross–bridge cycle in the myofibrils.

- There are several types of experimental evidence showing that central factors can limit muscle performance in certain situations. Nevertheless, there is even stronger evidence that peripheral factors, which directly affect contractile function, are of greater importance for muscle fatigue during resistance training.

- Overall, lactate appears to have a negligible effect on muscle fatigue.

- Accumulation of potassium around the muscle membrane is thought to contribute to muscle fatigue, but the evidence in the context of resistance training is unclear.

- Accumulation of inorganic phosphate ions has been shown to play an important role in muscle fatigue by leading to impaired cross–bridge function.

- The accumulation of phosphate ions is also the most important cause of impaired calcium release in the muscle cells, which is closely associated with muscle fatigue.

- Muscles with low glycogen levels fatigue faster than muscles with high glycogen levels, probably because impaired calcium balance occurs earlier when glycogen stores are low.

- Exercise–induced muscle damage (EIMD) triggers muscle soreness and impairs maximum strength.

- The time course of EIMD can range from almost immediate symptoms to effects that last at least a week after exercise.

- EIMD is most pronounced after exercises involving eccentric muscle actions.

- EIMD usually peaks between 24 and 48 hours after exercise and then gradually disappears over the following days.

- The inflammatory processes in the muscles follow approximately the same time course as muscle soreness.

- Reduced muscle function is greatest immediately after exercise and then gradually recovers.

- The "repeated–bout effect" refers to the notion that after an episode of EIMD, the muscle is better protected the next time it is subjected to a similar stress.

- During EIMD, micro damage to muscle fibers can be observed, especially around the Z–discs. There is also active protein breakdown of structural and contractile proteins.

- The perceived muscle soreness is likely due to an interaction between the micro damage to the muscle fibers, which causes cell swelling and immune cell infiltration into the damaged areas, and the impaired calcium balance in the fibers.

- There are several different methods that have been tested to reduce the symptoms of EIMD or speed recovery, but most are ineffective.

- Dietary polyphenols have been shown to have anti–inflammatory and antioxidant effects. The most promising evidence for a positive effect on recovery from EIMD comes from studies on pomegranates and tart cherries.

CHAPTER 14

RECOVERY STRATEGIES

Athletes and fitness enthusiasts use a number of strategies to speed up the recovery process between workouts, but do they work? In this chapter, we will examine some of the most commonly used recovery methods and their potential impact on the recovery process after resistance exercise.

COLD-WATER IMMERSION

Cold water immersion (CWI) or ice baths have become an increasingly popular recovery strategy for various sports. The goal is to stimulate blood flow and thereby speed recovery. The typical protocol involves immersing a larger portion of the body in cold water (often 10–15 C°) for 10–15 minutes. Research in this area has increased significantly over the past decade, focusing primarily on whether ice bathing accelerates performance recovery. The general conclusion from the review articles in this field is that ice baths can have a small positive effect on the recovery of e.g., muscle strength [247,248].

A Swedish study investigated performance recovery and muscle contractility during severe cooling compared with warming [249]. It was reported that cooling had a negative effect on recovery because glycogen stores were less replenished. However, the cooling protocol in this experiment was much more severe than in the usual ice bath protocols. The optimal protocol for CWI in terms of temperature and duration remains to be determined. It is possible that part of the beneficial effect noted in some studies is due to the placebo effect, as it is impossible to perform an ice bath blindly.

As CWIs for recovery become more popular, it has been investigated whether repeated ice baths can affect muscle adaptation to exercise. In general, no major effect was found on adaptations to endurance training, such as markers of mitochondrial biogenesis. As for adaptations to resistance training, there is emerging evidence that the development of muscle strength and hypertrophy may be affected by post-exercise ice baths. In a study published in 2015 from Australia, 21 subjects performed resistance training followed by a 10-minute ice bath or active recovery [250]. The group subjected to CWI had attenuated strength development and decreased muscle mass gains compared to the control group. Analysis of muscle biopsies revealed that the impaired training adaptations were associated with lower anabolic signaling and satellite cell activation. In addition, a recent study reported decreased myofibrillar protein synthesis after repeated ice baths during a resistance training program [251].

Recently, a growing number of professional athletes, as well as recreational athletes, have begun to explore whole-body cryotherapy, administered in specialized cryochambers, as a potential way to improve health and possibly promote muscle recovery and function. Despite the appeal of this high-tech approach, it is important to note that these devices tend to be expensive and that there is no convincing evidence to date that their effectiveness is significantly different from that of a traditional ice bath.

In summary, there is some evidence that cold water therapies may negatively influence muscle adaptations to resistance training. Because the effects on recovery are relatively modest, the overarching recommendation for athletes and individuals engaged in resistance training, especially those seeking optimal training adaptation, is that ice baths should be used with caution. Of course, there may be situations where the use of ice baths is warranted, such as during periods of intense training or frequent competition. In such cases, however, they should be considered a short-term strategy rather than a routine procedure.

ANTIOXIDANTS

Antioxidants are substances that neutralize free oxygen and nitrogen radicals (reactive oxygen species, ROS) in cells. Several nutrients in the diet act as antioxidants, such as vitamin E, vitamin C, coenzyme Q10, riboflavin and carotenoids. It has long been known that these antioxidants play an important role in the body, as high concentrations of free radicals can react with DNA and damage our cells. Physical activity increases our body's consumption of oxygen, which in turn increases the production of free radicals. Therefore, it has been suggested that physically active people should consume additional antioxidants, perhaps even through dietary supplements.

However, despite the increased ROS production during exercise, our cells have a very well-controlled system for dealing with free radicals. Most people consume enough antioxidants through their normal diet. In addition, regular exercise leads to improved antioxidant protection. In fact, antioxidants have been found to be detrimental to the adaptive response to exercise. This was first shown in studies on mice, but has now been shown in studies on humans, both in terms of adaptation to endurance training and to resistance training.

In a 10-week resistance training study, subjects received high doses of vitamins C and E or a placebo during the training period [252]. In the antioxidant group, decreased translational signaling (the process that initiates protein synthesis) and impaired strength development was reported. Thus, it appears that antioxidant supplementation can dampen the signal for training adaptations, likely because free radicals are involved in cell signaling that interacts with our genes and, ultimately, muscle protein turnover.

It is sometimes claimed that antioxidants speed up the recovery process after exercise. For many fitness enthusiasts, of course, it would be very tempting to use supplements that allow you to train harder. However, the scientific support for this is very weak. In the vast majority of studies, recovery of muscle function and exercise-induced muscle soreness are not affected by taking antioxidants [253].

One problem is that these supplements often contain very high doses of antioxidants, far in excess of daily requirements. Chronic intake of such high doses of antioxidants has been associated not only with impaired muscle adaptation, but also with an increased risk of all-cause mortality [254]. However, because these alarming results are from observational studies, a causal relationship has yet to be demonstrated.

ANTI-INFLAMMATORY DRUGS

Both elite and recreational athletes frequently take nonsteroidal anti-inflammatory drugs (NSAIDs, such as ibuprofen and diclofenac). These medications are taken by athletes to relieve pain or speed recovery after muscle soreness, injuries, or hard workouts. Although NSAIDs relieve pain and inflammation, there is little scientific evidence that these drugs affect performance, recovery, or exercise-induced muscle damage. If there is any effect at all, it tends to be small.

However, there is a risk that NSAIDs may have longer-term negative effects because the inflammatory response associated with acute exercise is an important signal for the synthesis of new muscle proteins and subsequent muscular adaptations. In this regard, it has been found that the use of over-the-counter NSAIDs can decrease muscle protein synthesis and satellite cell activation after a single bout of resistance exercise [255,256].

In the largest study examining the effects of NSAID use on adaptations to resistance training, relatively untrained subjects completed an 8-week training period while taking either a high dose of ibuprofen (1200 mg per day) or a low dose of aspirin (75 mg of acetylsalicylic acid per day) [257]. The results showed that although both groups increased muscle mass as a result of training, the hypertrophic response was significantly attenuated in the ibuprofen group. The differences in strength development were not as marked, but the ibuprofen group still improved less than the control group. There was no difference in exercise performance (lifted loads) between the groups.

Overall, the results showed that high doses of NSAIDs have a negative effect on both muscle hypertrophy and strength. The mechanisms explaining the large difference between the groups are not yet fully understood, but from the molecular analyzes performed, it appeared that molecular factors involved in the inflammatory response and protein degradation were affected by the high dose of NSAIDs [258]. This strengthens the hypothesis that exercise-induced inflammatory processes are an important component of the molecular machinery that ultimately leads to muscle hypertrophy in response to resistance training.

SPOTLIGHT
Are there risks in taking painkillers?
· ·

Taking NSAIDs or other pain medications, such as acetaminophen (paracetamol), unnecessarily is not recommended because it carries some risks and possible side effects. The most common side effects are gastrointestinal problems and in severe cases, bleeding ulcers. Because NSAIDs inhibit platelet function, the risk of bleeding increases, and the consequences of injury can be more severe. These drugs have also been shown to increase the risk of acute cardiovascular events in the elderly and sick, although this risk is small in absolute terms. Overdose is the most dangerous aspect of acetaminophen. Few nonprescription drugs have as narrow a range between effective and harmful doses as acetaminophen. Overdose poses the greatest risk of liver toxicity. There are, of course, a variety of circumstances that justify the use of analgesics, but regular use should be preceded by a careful risk–benefit analysis, preferably in consultation with medical professionals.

COMPRESSION GARMENTS

One recovery method that has become increasingly popular over the past decade is the use of various types of compression garments that apply light pressure to the muscles. The idea is that compression improves venous return and/or reduces swelling and muscle soreness associated with resistance training. A meta-analysis showed that compression garments may have a small positive effect on muscle strength recovery after resistance training, at least from 24 hours after training and beyond [259]. The effects on exercise–induced muscle soreness or inflammatory markers are generally quite small, and the studies to date are inconclusive. It also remains to be investigated whether compression garments, like several other recovery methods, may have negative effects on long–term training adaptations.

SUMMARY

- ➲ Ice baths or cold–water immersions (CWI), but also whole–body cryotherapy, have become increasingly popular as a recovery strategy.

- ➲ Ice baths can have a small positive effect on strength recovery.

- ➲ Both muscle hypertrophy and strength development can be attenuated by repeated ice baths in conjunction with resistance training.

- ➲ Athletes who wish to maximize their training adaptations should therefore use ice baths restrictively and use them only as a temporary measure during periods of intense training or competition.

- ➲ Physical exercise increases the body's oxygen consumption and thus the production of free radicals (reactive oxygen species).

- ➲ However, regular exercise leads to improved antioxidant protection.

- ➲ High intake of antioxidant supplements may impair muscle adaptations to resistance training.

- There is limited scientific evidence that antioxidants can speed recovery or reduce exercise-induced muscle soreness.

- The general recommendation is to consume antioxidants through a balanced diet rather than supplements.

- Athletes and recreational athletes often take non-steroidal anti-inflammatory drugs (NSAIDs).

- NSAIDs do not appear to speed recovery or reduce exercise-induced muscle soreness.

- NSAIDs can attenuate muscle protein synthesis and impair satellite cell activation after resistance exercise.

- In young adults, there is evidence that NSAIDs may attenuate muscle hypertrophy and strength gains.

- Compression garments may have a small positive effect on muscle recovery after resistance training. However, the long-term consequences for muscle adaptation to exercise have not yet been investigated.

CHAPTER 15

CONCURRENT RESISTANCE AND ENDURANCE TRAINING

There seems to be a perception among many that performing endurance and resistance training simultaneously could potentially compromise muscle hypertrophy and strength gains. However, this notion is generally overstated. Significant improvements in strength and muscle mass can be achieved with concurrent strength and endurance training, and resistance training often has a positive effect on endurance performance. Nevertheless, there may be some scenarios in which these opposing training modalities do not work well together. In this chapter, we will take a closer look at the controversial topic of concurrent training and the related phenomenon of the "interference effect".

BACKGROUND TO RESEARCH ON CONCURRENT TRAINING

Specific adaptations occur in both athletes and recreational athletes who engage in prolonged and regular resistance or endurance training. These adaptations result in a phenotype that reflects the predominant form of training. To illustrate, consider the different muscle composition of marathon runners and bodybuilders. The marked difference is a practical, if somewhat extreme, example of how different the endurance and strength phenotypes can be, and likely demonstrates that combining resistance and endurance training can be challenging. It would be inconceivable for a bodybuilder to adopt the training program of a marathon runner and still expect a steady improvement in muscle mass. This underscores the importance of specific training in achieving desired performance results in a particular sport or physical endeavor.

Classic adaptations of muscles to endurance training include morphological and metabolic changes such as increased mitochondrial and capillary density and higher concentrations of oxidative enzymes that lead to improved endurance performance. In contrast, as has become clear in the previous chapters of this book, resistance training leads to muscle hypertrophy and increased strength.

Thus, strength and endurance training lead to different muscular adaptations that are often considered opposites. However, there is a large overlap between these extremes. For example, both muscle and fiber size can increase in response to endurance training, and changes in fiber type composition are often in the same direction regardless of the type of training. In addition, resistance training may lead to increased formation of new capillaries, which is traditionally attributed to endurance training. These examples illustrate that the adaptive response to exercise is complex and occurs along a continuum.

The first study on this topic was published by Robert Hickson in 1980 [260]. The anecdote is that after a run with his mentor, he began to wonder if the muscle could really adapt to strength and endurance training simultaneously. Hickson's study compared three groups: Resistance training alone, combined resistance and endurance training, or endurance training alone 5–6 days per week for 10 weeks. The resistance training group and the combined group showed similar strength improvements (1RM squats) by week 7 (Fig. 15.1). Thereafter, strength continued to increase in the resistance training–only group, while the progress of the combined training group deteriorated in the last three weeks. This study laid the foundation for future research on concurrent training, and the idea that endurance training interferes with strength development was born.

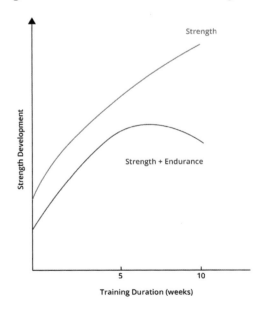

Figure 15.1.
Strength development during 10 weeks of resistance training alone compared with combined resistance and endurance training. Based on data from Hickson 1980. The complete reference can be found in the Figure references section at the end of the book.

EFFECTS OF CONCURRENT TRAINING ON MUSCLE HYPERTROPHY

Since the number of concurrent training studies has become quite large, but the studies are generally quite small, it is important to look at the studies that have examined all the research on muscle hypertrophy with concurrent training versus resistance training alone. A recent meta–analysis showed that there is no overall interference effect of endurance training on muscle hypertrophy [261]. However, the effect appears to be dependent on the specific design of the training program. Of the few studies that have shown a negative effect of endurance training on muscle hypertrophy, none have determined muscle size by MRI or CT. Instead, the degree of hypertrophy was assessed by measuring fiber size from biopsies taken before and after the training period. This measurement technique is subject to large methodological errors, so it may be problematic to draw conclusions from fiber data based on 7–8 individuals in each training group (as was often the case).

Program design factors

In evaluating the potential effects of different endurance training modalities, it appears that running may have a more detrimental effect on muscle fiber hypertrophy than cycling [262]. However, it is important to note that only a limited number of studies have included running as an endurance training modality and that the observations to date have been mainly on muscle fiber size rather than whole muscle size. This is consistent with a discovery by de Souza et al. who examined both fiber size and whole muscle adaptations [263]. Interestingly, they were unable to demonstrate any impairment of muscle hypertrophy at the level of the whole muscle, but only at the level of the fibers.

The observation that running potentially exacerbates the interference effect in type I fibers compared to cycling could be due to the unique characteristics of the two activities. Running, which involves repetitive eccentric loading and stretch–shortening actions, differs from cycling, which focuses more on concentric work and allows for longer time under tension. This difference may lead to increased inflammatory and catabolic stress induced by running compared to cycling.

There are numerous training variables that could influence the hypertrophy response to concurrent training, including factors such as training frequency, training status, exercise modality, and the order of exercise within the same session. However, in the recent meta–analysis, none of these aspects proved to be a significant moderator of the effect of concurrent training on hypertrophy. It is important to note that most studies were conducted with relatively moderate training volumes. There is a plausible assumption that optimal adaptation may become more difficult at high frequencies and/or volumes of concurrent training. In addition, most of the studies conducted were of short duration, i.e., 12 weeks or less. It is plausible that optimal adaptation to divergent training methods over longer periods of time could be more challenging, especially for individuals who are already well–trained.

Another variable to consider is the order of the different types of training and whether they are scheduled on the same or alternate days within a training week. To date, this factor does not appear to have a significant effect on the development of muscle hypertrophy with concurrent training.

Proposed interference mechanisms

Despite the general lack of studies clearly demonstrating that the interference effect in relation to muscle hypertrophy exists at all, there have been several attempts to explore it using different approaches. The high metabolic stress associated with endurance training may activate signaling pathways that reduce muscle protein synthesis [264]. Thus, while performing resistance training prior to endurance training ensures high quality during resistance training, the subsequent endurance stimuli may still decrease the anabolic response of the muscle.

A very attractive hypothesis was presented in the mid–2000s. It was based on animal experiments showing that strength and endurance training activate different cellular signaling pathways that are specific to the exercise stimuli. Resistance training activates the mTOR signaling cascade, which leads to increased synthesis of contractile proteins, whereas endurance training stimulates the AMPK/PGC–1α signaling cascade, which ultimately stimulates mitochondrial biogenesis [265]. Therefore, because increased myofibrillar protein synthesis in response to resistance training is central to muscle hypertrophy, endurance training has been hypothesized to impair muscle growth and strength development by reducing muscle protein synthesis.

However, in a series of human studies examining the effects of endurance training on molecular, functional, and muscular adaptations to resistance training after both acute and chronic training, the results showed that mTOR signaling was stronger after concurrent training than after resistance training alone, and muscle hypertrophy was also more pronounced after concurrent training [61,266]. One of the studies examined the effects of concurrent endurance and resistance training before and after a 5–week training period in which the training sessions were separated by a recovery period of only 15 minutes. Despite the short recovery period and the fact that AMPK was activated after endurance training, 5 weeks of concurrent training still resulted in a greater increase in muscle volume than resistance training alone [267].

While the fatigue and metabolic stress associated with endurance exercise did not affect the hypertrophic response to subsequent resistance training in this study, the development of concentric strength was attenuated by the preceding endurance training, suggesting that short periods of rest between training sessions negatively affect strength development. Recovery to restore muscle function between training sessions is therefore important to achieve maximal strength and power development, which we will discuss below.

EFFECTS OF CONCURRENT TRAINING ON MAXIMAL STRENGTH AND POWER

The compatibility of concurrent resistance and endurance training with the development of maximal and explosive strength is important to examine for those who want to perform endurance training while maximizing the benefits of resistance training. Several studies suggest that endurance training may limit the development of maximal strength, isokinetic force production, explosive strength, and vertical jump performance [268]. However, at the meta–analysis level, the effect on maximal strength is not significant when all studies are considered together [261]. The main moderating variable for maximum strength appears to be training status, where trained individuals may note a small interference effect on the development of maximum strength compared to untrained or moderately trained individuals [269].

The negative effect of concurrent strength and endurance training on explosive strength was corroborated in a meta–analysis [261]. Interestingly, this effect was particularly pronounced when the exercise types were performed simultaneously in the same session. However, when the training sessions were at least three hours apart, the negative effect on explosive strength was no longer significant. It is reasonable to assume that the potentially negative effect of endurance training on strength development is amplified by high training volume and fatigue, which may affect the quality of subsequent training sessions [270].

Mechanisms for impaired explosive strength

Since concurrent training does not seem to affect hypertrophy in general, it is important to investigate other mechanisms that could explain the observed impairment of explosive strength. Among the proposed mechanisms underlying the negative effect on explosive strength with concurrent training, decreased neural activation emerges as an important explanation.

A 2003 Finnish research study provides valuable insight into this phenomenon. In this study, individuals were combining resistance and endurance training in a 20–week program [271]. After the training period, the participants failed to improve rapid neural activation at the onset of maximal contraction, which is required to increase rate of force development. Upon closer inspection, it was found that although maximal neural activation remained unchanged, the increase in the integrated electromyographic signal during the first 500 milliseconds was attenuated in the group performing both endurance and resistance training.

Because the maximal rate of force development is largely determined by the rate of recruitment and maximal discharge of motor neurons, the data suggest that these processes are particularly susceptible to the interference effects of endurance training. It can be hypothesized that the residual fatigue induced by endurance training may interfere with the corticospinal inputs that motor neurons receive prior to force generation. This interference would subsequently affect rapid force generation, a crucial element in the process of explosive force generation. Such impairment could affect the quality of resistance training when performed concurrently with aerobic exercise and result in impaired development of explosive strength.

Order effect

Regarding the order of training sessions, it is often recommended to perform resistance training before endurance training if both modalities are to be trained on the same day. Indeed, high–intensity endurance training could reduce the quality of the subsequent resistance training [272,273], suggesting that the incompatibility between endurance and resistance training is minimized if resistance training is performed first [270].

However, it has also been reported that performing endurance training immediately after jump training decreases the improvement in maximal jumping power compared to jump training without additional training [274]. Thus, while it is advisable to recommend resistance training in a fresh and rested state, there is no guarantee that adaptations will be optimal if power–based training is immediately followed by endurance training.

Ultimately, the goal of the training session and the overall training plan must be considered when determining the order in which you will perform the various workouts. However, a general recommendation might be to separate endurance and resistance training sessions whenever possible.

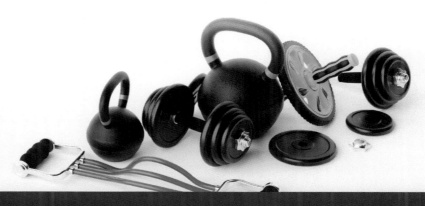

SPOTLIGHT
How can a concurrent training program be effectively designed?

It is challenging to formulate universal recommendations for concurrent training because the needs and requirements can vary greatly depending on the goal, training status, and specific characteristics of different sports. In addition, the training goal often evolves over different phases within an annual training plan, further complicating general guidelines. Therefore, an individualized approach to concurrent training program design is recommended, considering specific needs and contexts.

A pragmatic approach is to prioritize one physical capacity at a time in training and maintain the other by training it once or twice a week. This strategy is supported by evidence that a modest volume of strength or endurance training, when performed at high intensity, can be sufficient to not only maintain but possibly even improve the respective quality.

For recreational athletes and older individuals seeking to improve their overall fitness and health, the synergistic combination of resistance and endurance training should be appreciated and can provide complementary benefits. Conversely, athletes whose primary goal is to develop strength and explosiveness should allow adequate recovery time after endurance training before beginning resistance training.

In scenarios where endurance and resistance training are scheduled in the same training session, starting with resistance training could ensure a high training quality. If it is possible to split the training sessions, e.g., morning and afternoon or evening, endurance training could come first, allowing for a longer recovery period (at least overnight) after resistance training.

RESISTANCE TRAINING FOR ENDURANCE PERFORMANCE

A review of the research literature shows that well–designed resistance training can improve endurance performance [275]. However, only recently has the integration of resistance training into traditional endurance sports received the recognition and attention it rightly deserves. In the past, endurance athletes expressed reservations about resistance training because they feared possible weight gain. Such weight gain could pose a significant challenge, especially in endurance sports where the ability to efficiently carry one's body weight is an essential component of performance. However, concerns about weight gain from resistance training are unwarranted. In most studies in which resistance training was added to an endurance training program, body weight remained unchanged.

Although maximal oxygen uptake is not affected by the addition of resistance training, performance is usually improved. One of the most important explanations for the improvement in endurance performance with additional resistance training is that work economy is improved; the athlete simply uses less oxygen and energy at a given work intensity, for example, at a given speed on the treadmill. The mechanism that explains why resistance training can improve running economy is at least partially related to the increased stiffness of tendons and connective tissue that results from resistance training [276]. A stiffer tendon can store more energy when loaded, and this energy is returned in the subsequent shortening phase (the stretch–shortening cycle).

Indirect evidence for this effect is provided by cross–sectional data showing that the running economy of well–trained runners correlates negatively with performance in the sit–and–reach test [277], a flexibility test for the hamstring muscles on the back of the thigh (you sit with your legs extended on the ground and try to reach your toes).

In a study of elite orienteers in the late 1990s, it was shown that runners who replaced part of their endurance training with resistance training improved both 5-kilometer running performance, work economy, and ability to run at high speed when fatigued[278]; the control group, which maintained the traditional program, showed no improvement after the 9-week training period. In addition, resistance training has been shown to have positive effects on performance in sport-specific tests for cyclists and cross-country skiers[275,279], so there are good reasons for endurance athletes to review their allocation between endurance and resistance training in the training program.

In addition to improving work economy, resistance training can also lead to an increased ability to perform at high power outputs at the end of a race. Properly performed resistance training can also contribute to fewer injuries and better function in certain sports movements. Overall, resistance training should be considered for both elite and recreational athletes. The specific sport and the athlete's individual goals must determine how the specific resistance training program should be designed.

Tendon stiffness to improve work economy appears to be best trained in short but intense sessions that emphasize heavy weights and explosive actions. This can be combined with various types of jump training. If the goal is to improve performance in sport-specific actions, the principle of specificity applies, and one should preferably use sport-specific exercises while ensuring that great force development and maximal effort can be achieved in the selected exercises. Resistance training for athletes is discussed in more detail in Chapter 17.

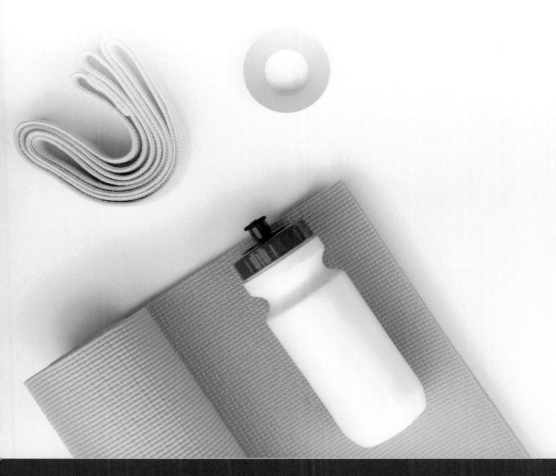

SUMMARY

- There are both similarities and distinct differences between muscular adaptations to traditional resistance and endurance training.

- The seminal study by Robert Hickson in 1980 established the concept of concurrent training. It showed similar strength improvements in strength–only and combined groups, but progress in the combined group deteriorated in the final weeks.

- A review of meta–analysis results shows no significant overall interference effect of endurance training on muscle hypertrophy, though results may be dependent on training design.

- Running appears to be more likely to impair muscle hypertrophy than cycling.

- High training frequency and high total training volume may increase the risk that endurance training will impair muscle hypertrophy.

- Several hypotheses have been investigated to understand the interference effect. These include the study of signaling pathways such as mTOR and AMPK/PGC–1α and the effect of metabolic stress associated with endurance training on muscle protein synthesis. However, there is little support for interference in muscle hypertrophy.

- Strength gains may be somewhat impaired when endurance training is added to the resistance training program. This risk of interference is greatest for explosive strength, and residual fatigue and closely spaced training sessions may increase the risk that endurance training will impair explosive strength.

- A practical recommendation for athletes might be to periodize training within different cycles so that one form of training is prioritized while the other form of training is performed at a maintenance level.

- Athletes who prioritize the development of strength and explosiveness should recover sufficiently after endurance training before performing resistance training and aim for a low total endurance training volume.

- Complementary and beneficial effects of concurrent endurance and resistance training are observed in recreational athletes training for better overall fitness and health.

- Resistance training is generally beneficial for endurance performance by improving work economy and the ability to rapidly increase and maintain a high power output.

CHAPTER 16

HEALTH BENEFITS OF RESISTANCE TRAINING

Resistance training, once associated mostly with athletes and bodybuilders, is now becoming a fundamental part of a healthy lifestyle that affects most organ systems of the human body. In the past, skepticism about resistance training was widespread. People feared possible risks and were unaware of the extensive physiological benefits it offers. In recent years, however, there has been a paradigm shift in the perception of resistance training, and its positive effects on health are increasingly recognized, and not just as a means of building muscle or improving appearance. This chapter looks at resistance training from a health perspective.

RESISTANCE TRAINING FOR HEALTH

It is difficult to argue against the well-known positive effects of physical activity and exercise on health. Observational studies show a strong relationship between physical activity levels and the risk of disease and premature death. Most of the research on physical activity and health has focused on aerobic exercise, which some would define as anything from avoiding a sedentary lifestyle to moderate to high intensity structured exercise. This is also reflected in physical activity guidelines in most countries around the world. Although they include a general recommendation to perform "muscle-strengthening activities" twice a week, the recommendations focus on physical activities of aerobic nature.

Recently, there has been a noticeable shift in emphasis toward recognizing the positive health benefits of resistance training. This shift is significant, especially considering that just a few decades ago, resistance training was primarily associated with bodybuilders and powerlifters. Today, we know that resistance training has a positive effect on several risk factors for disease. Resistance training also appears to correlate with a lower risk of premature death, regardless of cause (all-cause mortality) [280].

It is important to recognize that categorizing resistance training and endurance training as completely different types of training can sometimes be misleading from a health perspective. In fact, they often share many of the same health benefits [281]. Resistance training, when designed with a specific approach such as circuit training, can improve muscle strength and cardiovascular fitness simultaneously. This integrated focus on muscular and cardiovascular health is an example of the convergence between the two training modalities.

As discussed in the chapter on energy metabolism during resistance training, many conventional resistance training routines that use large muscle groups can be sufficiently demanding to meet the criteria for moderate intensity as prescribed in the physical activity guidelines. This provides an interesting perspective that blurs the traditional boundaries between these types of training and highlights that individual exercise sessions can fulfill the dual goals of muscle strengthening and aerobic conditioning.

The following are examples of several diseases, clinical conditions, or risk markers for which there is at least moderately strong evidence that resistance training has a beneficial effect, either directly against the disease/condition itself or indirectly through improved well-being and functional abilities, likely improving prognosis [282,283]:

- Lower back pain
- Cardiovascular disease
- Stroke
- Insulin resistance and type 2 diabetes
- Osteoporosis
- Hypertension (high blood pressure)
- Dyslipidemia
- Obesity
- Depression
- Dementia

- Parkinson
- MS
- Heart failure
- Chronic obstructive pulmonary disease
- Cystic fibrosis
- Arthritis
- Rheumatoid arthritis
- Cancer

Although this book does not address the specific details of various clinical conditions, it is important to understand that there are numerous beneficial health effects of exercise that are produced by the physiological response it elicits. Regardless of whether one is in a healthy or sick state, a physically active lifestyle that emphasizes both the cardiorespiratory system and skeletal muscles is probably the optimal way to benefit health.

High–intensity interval training (HIIT) is gaining recognition as a valuable method for promoting health. HIIT combines a lower training volume with high intensity, which affects both the cardiovascular system and skeletal muscle, especially in terms of metabolic effects.

This approach complicates the conventional distinction between endurance and resistance training as separate forms of exercise. While endurance and resistance training may represent extremes when viewed in isolation, the reality of modern fitness practice shows a blending of these categories. Factors such as volume, duration, intensity, and training frequency dictate the body's response, creating a spectrum of adaptations and effects rather than a dichotomy.

Nonetheless, among the various exercise modalities, resistance training is the most effective means of maintaining or increasing muscle mass and strength. It also improves functional abilities that are essential for performing daily tasks. Unfortunately, it has been reported that only one in five adults comply with the recommended guidelines and perform both aerobic exercise and muscle–strengthening activities [284]. Thus, large–scale public health initiatives appear to be important if the burden of non–communicable diseases is to be mitigated through improved fitness in the population.

RESISTANCE TRAINING AND CARDIOVASCULAR HEALTH

Physical activity and exercise are strongly associated with a lower risk of cardiovascular disease. Indeed, there is a dose–response relationship in which more physical activity is associated with an even greater reduction in risk [285]. While most of the evidence has come from studies of aerobic physical activity, it is increasingly recognized that similar health effects are seen with resistance training. High levels of muscular strength appear to be in themselves a marker of lower cardiovascular disease risk, being associated with lower incidence of chronic inflammation, insulin resistance, and obesity [286].

One risk factor for cardiovascular disease worth discussing is high blood pressure (hypertension). Research over the past decade has shown that resistance training can be as beneficial as traditional endurance training in lowering blood pressure. In particular, isometric hand–grip training appears to be very effective. In this form of exercise, the exerciser should tighten a hand dynamometer at about 50% of maximum force, maintain static tension for 1–2 minutes, and then repeat a few times per workout and a few times per week. Such training may be even more effective than endurance training in lowering resting blood pressure [287].

RESISTANCE TRAINING AND TYPE 2 DIABETES

Type 2 diabetes is a progressive disease associated with an increased risk of cardiovascular disease. The disease is defined by high plasma glucose levels due to insulin resistance and/or increasing insulin deficiency. Increased physical activity and other lifestyle interventions are considered fundamental to reducing insulin resistance. A single exercise session, regardless of modality, increases skeletal muscle glucose uptake primarily by increasing translocation of the glucose transporter GLUT–4, resulting in glucose being transported into the cell without insulin. Since this effect occurs only up to 24–48 hours after exercise, it is recommended to exercise regularly to achieve long–term positive blood glucose control.

A combination of endurance and resistance exercise has been shown to have the best effect on plasma glucose control and is therefore recommended [288]. However, resistance training has beneficial effects even without endurance training. Both high intensity and long duration of exercise are considered beneficial for glycemic control, and high intensity may partially compensate for a shorter duration. However, for optimal effect, exercise should be performed regularly (at least every other day) and involve large muscle groups.

RESISTANCE TRAINING FOR SPECIFIC PATIENT GROUPS

Interest in resistance training as a supplement or adjunct to traditional treatment of various diseases has increased recently. Recent research has shown that cancer patients undergoing chemotherapy can perform resistance training with positive effects [289]. In this study, patients with breast cancer were evaluated for the effects of different types of exercise on fatigue, physical performance, cancer–specific symptoms, physical function, and muscle structure and function before and immediately after chemotherapy and one year later. The results showed that women who performed resistance training and high–intensity interval training became less tired, less sensitive to pain, and stronger. Training also had a positive effect on fitness, body weight, and cancer–related symptoms, and led to specific muscle–level adaptations, such as maintaining fiber size, compared with general impairments in the control group [290].

There is a growing body of evidence that resistance training also has beneficial effects, for example, in post–stroke rehabilitation, heart failure, chronic pain conditions, multiple sclerosis, rheumatoid arthritis, osteoarthritis, back and neck pain, and Parkinson's disease, to name a few. There are very few, if any, chronic diseases for which resistance training should be avoided, and the restrictions usually apply only to a specific phase of the disease. However, various acute conditions such as unstable coronary artery disease, severe aortic stenosis, uncontrolled cardiac arrhythmias, acute myocardial infarction, pulmonary embolism, or very high blood pressure (>200/115 mm Hg) are still considered absolute contraindications to any form of strenuous physical activity [291].

RESISTANCE TRAINING AND COGNITIVE FUNCTION

Various aspects of cognitive function tend to deteriorate with aging, which in turn has negative implications for individual health and independence. Systematic reviews have concluded that resistance training can have beneficial effects on several aspects of cognitive function, not least the ability to plan and perform tasks in everyday life (executive function) [292]. Memory may also be improved, although such effects are less clear in the literature. In certain conditions, such as stroke, resistance training for as little as 12 weeks can result in an improved ability to perform specific tasks and improve working memory and information processing [293]. The mechanisms explaining how resistance training can improve cognitive function are not fully understood, and as with many other outcome variables, there is wide variation in effects between different individuals.

RESISTANCE TRAINING AND BONE HEALTH

Many forms of resistance training result in positive effects on skeletal bone. Bone health is often assessed by measuring bone mineral density with DXA. Low bone mineral density is an important marker for the clinical diagnosis of osteoporosis, which affects approximately 30 million people in Europe [294] and 40 million in the US [295].

Osteoporosis is much more common in women than in men, largely due to decreased estrogen production after menopause. However, bone integrity is controlled not only by bone mineral density but also by factors such as microarchitecture, geometry, and bone turnover. In osteoporosis, there is an increased risk of bone fractures and serious consequences in the event of falls. Osteoporosis therefore has many similarities to sarcopenia (loss of muscle mass and function) in terms of risk factors and potential adverse health effects.

As mentioned in Chapter 9, to be effective, resistance training should provide a mechanical load to the skeleton to strengthen bones. Therefore, loads that provide greater mechanical stimulation than walking, cycling, or swimming, are recommended. Resistance training is therefore an excellent way to improve bone health. Studies show that people who do resistance training or weight-bearing activities have higher bone mass and bone mineral density than age-matched untrained people [296].

Because of the relatively low turnover of bone tissue, the effects of exercise on bone are not as great as on muscle. However, prolonged exercise interventions show that it is possible to increase bone mineral density by about 1–3% per year, even in the elderly [296]. The causal effect of resistance training on reducing the risk of fractures is difficult to investigate with intervention studies, but observational studies suggest that the risk is reduced [297]. However, it is difficult to say whether this is due to improved bone strength per se or simply to a reduced risk of falls. Regardless, it seems safe to say that muscle- and bone-strengthening activities, along with balance training, reduce the risk of fall-related accidents and fractures [298].

RESISTANCE TRAINING FOR WEIGHT LOSS

It is often argued that physical activity and resistance training are important in the fight against overweight and obesity. The logical background of this argument is that obesity occurs when energy intake exceeds energy expenditure over a long period of time. Thus, in theory, weight gain can be slowed, or weight loss can be induced by either reducing energy intake or increasing energy expenditure. Although this reasoning is correct in terms of energy balance, research shows that high energy intake is a greater contributor to the prevalence of obesity today than low energy expenditure. Similarly, restricting caloric intake is a more effective method of weight loss than attempting to increase energy expenditure through more physical activity.

SPOTLIGHT
Is physical activity ineffective in changing energy balance?

. . . .

The reasons why physical activity alone is not very effective as a method of weight loss may in part be related to the fact that we tend to compensate for physical activity either by increasing energy intake or by being sedentary during the remaining hours of the day [299]. There also appears to be an adaptive component in resting energy expenditure that essentially "beats back" weight loss [300]. Thus, the long-term effect of increased physical activity on daily energy expenditure is marginal. However, physical activity and exercise are associated with a greater ability of individuals to maintain their weight after weight loss, and because overall health effects are also achieved, physical activity, including resistance training, is recommended for anyone trying to lose weight [301].

Physical activity in general and resistance training in particular can be of great importance in achieving a more positive body composition. The relative distribution between fat and muscle in the body is an important health marker and is often of greater importance to health and various risk factors for disease than the weight itself or the weight–to–height ratio (body mass index, BMI).

Contrary to what is often claimed, it is possible to lose weight while maintaining or even increasing muscle mass [302]. The reason why this is possible is that protein balance and body fat balance are largely regulated by different mechanisms. Whether body fat is stored as triglycerides or broken down into free fatty acids is largely determined by energy balance. Thus, a caloric deficit leads to fat loss, while a caloric surplus leads to fat storage.

The protein balance of skeletal muscle is primarily determined by the amount of protein ingested and the amount of physical activity and exercise. The reason muscle mass may be lost in a caloric deficit is primarily because protein synthesis decreases [303]. However, resistance training and high protein intake counteract this decrease in protein synthesis and result in muscle mass being maintained or increasing.

To prove the principle, a study asked young men to consume either 1.2 or 2.4 grams of protein per kg of body weight over a 4–week period with reduced caloric intake (–40%). In addition, all subjects completed resistance training and high–intensity interval training 6 times per week. The results showed that the group with normal protein intake (1.2 grams) maintained their muscle mass, while the group that consumed 2.4 grams of protein gained fat–free mass by 1.2 kg during those 4 weeks [302]. Interestingly, the group with the high protein intake also lost more fat mass than the group that consumed the lower amount of protein. So, to successfully lose fat mass while maintaining or increasing muscle mass, you should do resistance training (preferably in combination with other types of training) and have a high protein intake.

SUMMARY

- ⮑ Just like endurance training, resistance training has positive effects on a variety of chronic diseases and risk factors for poor health.

- ⮑ All people, young, adult, and old, are recommended to do resistance training at least twice a week.

- ⮑ Resistance training is associated with a lower risk of cardiovascular disease and type 2 diabetes.

- ⮑ Isometric resistance training has positive effects on blood pressure.

- ⮑ Resistance training has a positive effect on health status for various chronic diseases.

- ⮑ One of the most important health effects of resistance training is the increase in muscle mass and strength, which increases the ability to maintain a high level of physical function as we age, while decreasing the risk of fall accidents.

- ⮑ Resistance training can improve cognitive function.

- ⮑ Resistance training has positive effects on bone integrity and density.

- ⮑ Resistance training reduces the risk of osteoporosis and bone fractures.

- ⮑ For weight loss, changes in diet are probably more important than changes in physical activity levels, but the recommendation is still to combine reduced energy intake with increased physical activity and resistance training.

- ⮑ Resistance training combined with high protein intake allows muscle mass to be maintained or increased while fat mass decreases during weight loss. This leads to a more favorable body composition.

CHAPTER 17

RESISTANCE TRAINING FOR SPECIFIC TARGET GROUPS

The motivations for resistance training can vary widely. Some people perform resistance training to achieve specific performance goals, while others seek to enjoy health benefits, change body composition, or promote general well–being. Just as training goals vary, so can the physiology of resistance training across different populations. This chapter discusses the physiology of resistance training for specific target populations such as children, the elderly, and athletes. It also examines resistance training during pregnancy and sex differences between men and women in response to resistance training.

RESISTANCE TRAINING FOR THE ELDERLY

The aging process is accompanied by a decrease in muscle mass and strength. This age-related loss of muscle mass and function is called sarcopenia. Because skeletal muscle contains about half of the human body's total protein pool, muscle wasting is a serious problem that has significant effects on important regulatory functions such as energy metabolism, immune system response, and temperature regulation. Because muscle is the largest source of protein available, it could also serve as an important reservoir of water and energy substances during extreme exercise.

The term sarcopenia comes from the Greek "sarx" and "penia," roughly meaning "loss of flesh". There is no single definition of sarcopenia, but one of the most widely accepted comes from the European Working Group on Sarcopenia and reads:

> "A syndrome characterized by progressive and generalized loss of skeletal muscle mass and strength with a risk of adverse outcomes such as physical disability, poor quality of life and death" [304]

As can be seen from the definition, both muscle mass and strength are affected, and loss of strength is the most important diagnostic factor nowadays. The proportion of individuals who can be classified as clinically sarcopenic increases rapidly after age 70, and after age 80, nearly half of all individuals can be classified as sarcopenic.

It should be noted that these figures are very rough because there is no single, globally accepted method for classifying sarcopenia and the reported incidence varies widely. A major problem is also that current methods have difficulty accounting for body size. This results in small and thin people being classified as sarcopenic much more often than people with a larger body size and people who are overweight. A solution to this problem could be the use of population Z-scores, where muscle values are expressed in relation to people with the same appearance (sex, height, and BMI). Indeed, this method has been applied using muscle-specific z-scores from MRI images, showing a successful adjustment for body size and a more appropriate classification of adverse muscle composition [305].

As life expectancy continues to increase in society, sarcopenia is likely to be a major problem for the healthcare system in the future. Already today, sarcopenia is associated with illness, institutionalization, loss of autonomy, decreased quality of life, and even death. The financial consequences for society are therefore significant.

Muscle mass generally begins to decline after age 30 to 40, and then declines at a rate of up to 0.5% per year until age 60-70 [306], after which a more dramatic loss often occurs. It is important to note that these data are based on cross-sectional studies comparing populations of different ages. Longitudinal data are scarce. Therefore, the trajectories of muscle loss with age presented in the literature are snapshots and do not provide information about individual trajectories over a lifetime. Certainly, there are people who lose very little muscle mass, and the dramatic increase in muscle loss with age is caused to some extent by people with health problems. A favorable genetic predisposition and regular exercise training can certainly help preserve both muscle mass and function as we age.

Nowadays, a distinction is often made between primary and secondary sarcopenia. Primary sarcopenia is the loss of muscle mass and function related to the aging process itself. Secondary sarcopenia is the accelerated muscle loss associated with aggravating circumstances such as disease, inactivity, and poor nutrition.

The causes of sarcopenia are probably multifactorial. The best-known factors contributing to sarcopenia can be summarized as follows [307]:

- ➲ Neuromuscular degeneration
- ➲ Changes in protein turnover and satellite cell function
- ➲ Changes in hormone levels and sensitivity to hormones
- ➲ Chronic inflammation and oxidative stress
- ➲ Lifestyle factors

Neuromuscular degeneration

Neuromuscular degeneration with age includes muscle atrophy, especially of fast type 2 fibers, loss of motor units, increased fat infiltration, and decreased ability to activate muscles neurally. The loss of motor neurons leads to a loss of innervation of muscle fibers and subsequently to fiber atrophy. A compensatory mechanism for this phenomenon is the reinnervation of other motor units. The fibers that have lost their connection to a neuron can be innervated by a new neuron. Although this process is active in aging muscles, it is not sufficient to completely prevent muscle atrophy. However, this mechanism is better developed in older people who are more resistant to aging-induced muscle atrophy [308].

Muscle wasting affects different muscle groups to varying degrees, but is most severe in type 2 fibers and somewhat greater in the legs than in the arms. Loss of muscle mass is also associated with decreased fascicle length and pennation angle, which are important for contractility [12]. Thus, several different factors contribute to decreased muscle function with age, including atrophy, loss of muscle fibers, and structural changes.

Protein turnover and satellite cell function

Net muscle protein turnover is determined by the balance between protein synthesis and breakdown. Dietary intake of essential amino acids serves as an important signal for increased protein synthesis. However, this sensitivity to amino acids decreases with age, a condition known as anabolic resistance. This results in an impaired ability to activate the molecular signals that control protein synthesis.

In addition, protein degradation systems, such as the ubiquitin-proteasome system, are turned on to a greater extent. Older people also show less activation of satellite cells in response to resistance training compared to young people [121]. All in all, several mechanisms appear to explain the diminishing response to anabolic stimuli in old age that contribute to net muscle breakdown in old age.

Hormones

Our hormone profile changes as we age. The levels of primary sex hormones (testosterone in men and estrogen in women) and growth hormone decrease, especially in women. These changes contribute to altered body composition, including an increase in visceral fat and a decrease in lean mass and bone mineral density [307]. Growth hormone therapy in the elderly to counteract muscle loss has not been shown to be effective. However, estrogen therapy in women is generally associated with improved maintenance of muscle mass after menopause (more on this later in this chapter).

Aging is also associated with increased cortisone levels, which may contribute to changes in body composition and cognitive function [309]. Many older people are also less sensitive to insulin. However, it is unclear whether this is due to aging itself or to other causes such as obesity, decreased physical activity, changes in diet, and low-grade chronic inflammation.

Chronic inflammation and oxidative stress

Many of the typical inflammatory markers, such as TNF–α, IL–6, and CRP, are elevated in the elderly population. This is commonly referred to as chronic low–grade inflammation. Several studies have found an association between systemic inflammation and sarcopenia. The increased inflammation contributes to both increased protein breakdown and decreased protein synthesis due to anabolic resistance.

Aging is also associated with increased oxidative stress, which is the production of reactive oxygen species. The age–related production of free radicals in muscle may be due to the decreased mitochondrial function often seen in older age [310]. Ultimately, increased oxidative stress may lead to increased protein degradation and decreased protein synthesis. Thus, increased inflammation and oxidative stress have very similar effects on skeletal muscle during aging; they both contribute to negative muscle protein turnover.

Lifestyle factors

Physical activity and a healthy diet are both important lifestyle factors that can slow age–related loss of muscle mass. In fact, some older people lose little muscle mass, and muscle mass can certainly be gained even in advanced age if resistance training is practiced. Physical activity recommendations for the elderly advocate at least 150 minutes of moderate–intensity physical activity per week and muscle–strengthening activities at least twice per week.

There is no question that structured resistance training is necessary to optimize muscle mass preservation in the elderly. Adequate levels of muscle mass and strength may also be important in the presence of illness or injury. The goal should be to remain above the functional threshold required to perform desired daily activities. A higher baseline is therefore protective against disability caused by involuntary episodes of inactivity and/or muscle wasting (Fig. 17.1).

Figure 17.1.
Muscle loss during aging (sarcopenia). The figure shows a hypothetical scenario in which the muscle loss that accompanies normal aging can be slowed by resistance training. This could postpone the age threshold at which you can no longer perform all daily activities. This increases the number of "functional years" and improves the chances of coping well with episodes of illness and inactivity that inevitably lead to impaired muscle function.

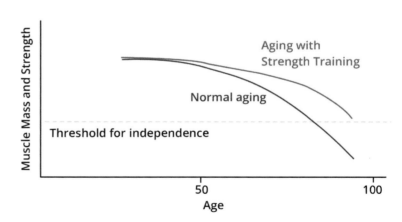

In a study of old Swedish skiers who had been physically active all their lives, exceptional working capacity and good health were found [311], yet muscle mass was no greater than in age–matched healthy controls. This supports the thesis that older people should engage in resistance training regardless of the volume of other types of physical activity.

This also raises the question: When is it too late to start? In fact, excellent results from resistance training have been noted even in 90–year–olds. After 8 weeks of training, Maria Fiatarone and her co–authors reported an amazing 174% increase in strength, while quadriceps muscle volume increased by 9% in ten frail, institutionalized volunteers [82]. In addition, walking speed increased by 48%. This clearly proves that even very old people benefit from resistance training.

A nutritional measure that could improve muscle mass preservation is to increase daily protein intake. Both protein intake and total energy intake often decrease with age [312]. This may be due to decreased appetite, deteriorated odor and taste, changes in the gastrointestinal tract, disease, or changes in the social environment. Adequate protein intake from a muscle maintenance perspective is about 1.2–1.6 g/kg of body weight per day, which is higher than what is currently recommended for the general population [313].

RESISTANCE TRAINING FOR CHILDREN AND ADOLESCENTS

There is little doubt that muscle and bone strengthening activities should be done at a young age. Several countries recommend that children and adolescents between the ages of 6 and 17 perform muscle- and bone-strengthening activities at least three times a week. Such activities can be performed as part of regular play, running, and jumping. Aside from the benefits to motor skills, physical development, and fitness, there is also preliminary evidence that muscular fitness and participation in resistance training are associated with better academic performance in school-aged youth [314].

The question of whether structured resistance training is beneficial or harmful for children and adolescents has sparked an unnecessarily polarized debate. For a long time, many organizations were restrictive in recommending resistance training for children. There were concerns that bone growth could be disrupted by damaging growth zones and that the risk of back problems could increase. These concerns also have some limited support in the literature. For example, back problems are common in some sports [315], but this is likely due to the stress of the sport itself and not the amount or type of resistance training.

The research literature generally emphasizes that resistance training is associated with a number of positive effects in children, including improved motor skills, increased strength, and decreased risk of injury. In fact, some advocates recommend starting systematic resistance training as early as 7–8 years of age. The addition of resistance training to traditional sport-specific training for adolescents can lead to improved performance on a number of different tests relevant to athletic performance [316]. The idea that resistance training at a young age can prevent injury is often highlighted as one of the most important benefits of resistance training for children and adolescents [317,318]. Here are some of the reported benefits of resistance training in children and adolescents listed:

- Increased perceived physical competence
- Self-confidence
- Increased strength and power
- Reduced risk of injury
- Increased spontaneous physical activity at school
- Combination with aerobic exercise can reduce fat mass
- Improved bone health

Although resistance training is generally considered safe, it is important to know that accidents are more common in children and adolescents than in adults [319]. In fact, injuries due to mishaps such as dropping weights or trying to lift weights that are too heavy are not negligible. Therefore, children should always be supervised and properly educated about the potential risks and proper handling of external weights. Emphasis must be placed on proper technique and execution. The overall focus should be on motor skills and overall physical development, not just performance and heavy lifting.

The risks of damage to bone structures and joints generally appear to be low and can often be attributed to accidents and poor technique [318]. It should be noted, however, that relatively few studies have examined the effects of long–term intensive resistance training in children and adolescents, and it would not be ethically permissible to design studies in which an immediate risk of injury may be suspected.

Even before puberty, children can make significant strength gains with systematic training [320]. Much of this strength gain is due to learning effects rather than muscular adaptation, although muscle growth does occur in children who engage in resistance training [321]. A meta–analysis examining the effects of resistance training in young girls (8–18 years) found that the positive effects were more pronounced in older girls (>15 years) than in younger [322]. This was confirmed in a meta–analysis including studies on both boys and girls, which found that the ability to gain muscle strength appears to increase with age and maturity status, and that the duration of the training program and the number of sets performed have a positive effect on the outcome [323].

The pubertal growth spurt is a phase characterized by a rapid increase in stature and muscle mass, especially in boys. Although girls usually enter puberty 1 to 2 years earlier than boys, the timing of the growth spurt can vary greatly from person to person. During puberty, the growth spurt and accompanying physical changes can have both positive and negative effects on performance. For example, there may be a period of adolescent awkwardness during which coordination decreases, and there is also a higher risk for growth–related injuries [324]. In addition, the increase in fat mass in girls can have a negative impact on certain performance metrics.

Overall, however, the effects of puberty on physical abilities tend to be positive. Strength performance and coordination are generally improved with resistance training, and after the growth spurt, the hypertrophic response to resistance training is generally improved. Thus, resistance training can be a valuable tool to address the various challenges of adolescence. However, it should be used with caution and tailored to the individual's needs and developmental stages. Careful consideration of these factors can help prevent injury and ensure that training is compatible with the growth and maturation of the young athlete.

In summary, structured resistance training for children and adolescents has both benefits and potential risks. It is important to ensure that resistance training is performed in a safe and proper manner with appropriate intensity/load. The focus should be on motor skills, technique, and athletic development rather than the pursuit of specific performance improvements at an early age. Thus, resistance training can be used as part of a varied, stimulating, and engaging training plan in children's and youth sports.

SEX ASPECTS IN RESISTANCE TRAINING

There is a considerable body of research that has examined biological sex differences in physiology, performance, and adaptations to resistance training. However, such studies present methodological challenges because they involve comparisons between two different groups where individual differences in training responses are large and there are obvious group differences at baseline. Because men tend to have greater muscle mass and are stronger than women, it can be difficult to determine whether the differences in exercise responses are sex–dependent or whether different baseline levels determine the magnitude of the changes.

Men have about 45% more lean body mass than women. The difference in muscle mass is more pronounced in the upper body muscles [325]. The sex difference in muscle strength is even greater, ranging from 40 to 120% depending on the exercise and muscle group studied [326]. Again, the differences are greater in the upper body. Even with the same muscle size, men have a significant strength advantage compared to women [327].

Regarding differences in muscle composition, women generally have slightly more intramuscular fat and thus a lower relative proportion of myofibrillar proteins. Women also rarely have larger type 2 fibers compared with type 1 fibers [328,329], which is otherwise relatively consistently the case in men. This results in a larger area fraction of type 1 fibers compared to type 2 fibers in females compared to males [15]. The information on fiber morphology is based mainly on biopsies from the vastus lateralis muscle on the thigh. It is not certain whether this is also true for other muscle groups or for highly trained populations.

When examining adaptations to resistance training, studies comparing men and women are often of limited size. Therefore, it is more informative to look at meta-analyzes that quantify the overall effect sizes of multiple studies. From this broader perspective, it appears that both men and women build muscle mass (hypertrophy) at the same relative rate, as measured by percent change [101].

Furthermore, both sexes increase strength at similar rates, although the relative increase in the upper body appears to be slightly more pronounced in women. This discrepancy raises interesting questions: Is the observed difference the result of a biological difference in training response or does it simply reflect a lower baseline and consequently a greater margin for improvement in women? To date, the cause of this difference remains unclear.

It is important to recognize that some of the differences between men and women in resistance training are not only physical, but could also be influenced by psychological or social factors. As James Nuzzo reports in a comprehensive review [326], men's motivation often lies in aspects such as challenge, competition, social recognition, and the pursuit of greater muscle mass and strength. This tendency leads them to prefer high-intensity exercises, upper-body exercises, and a competitive environment. In contrast, women's motivation often revolves around improving attractiveness, toning muscles, and weight management. They tend to be more inclined toward supervised lower body exercises. These contrasting motivations and preferences highlight that sex differences in resistance training may be shaped by societal norms and individual goals as well as physiological differences.

One of the most obvious differences between males and females is the level of sex hormones. At age 17, boys have about 30-40% more muscle mass than girls, which is related to a marked difference in testosterone levels that can be up to 20 times higher in boys than girls during puberty and persists into adulthood [330]. During resistance training, testosterone levels increase slightly in women compared with men acutely after exercise [331]. To date, however, there is no clear evidence that differences in exercise-induced hormonal responses control muscular adaptation to training. This is despite the fact that exogenous testosterone treatment can strongly influence protein synthesis in women [332].

In a study examining anabolic signaling and protein synthesis in men and women after a single bout of resistance training, no sex difference was found in the relative increase in protein synthesis, although the increase in testosterone was different [333]. Thus, it appears that the natural increase in endogenous hormone levels that occurs in association with resistance training does not regulate protein synthesis. Further evidence in support of the hypothesis that circulating testosterone does not cause sex differences in exercise responses is the fact that the basal protein turnover of skeletal muscle is comparable in women and men despite differences in hormone levels [334].

SPOTLIGHT
Can estrogen have anabolic effects?
· · · · · · · · · · · · · · · · · · · ·

Although hormone levels naturally fluctuate in women during the menstrual cycle, there is no evidence that short-term fluctuations in sex hormones during the menstrual cycle appreciably affect acute exercise performance or longer-term strength or hypertrophy adaptation to resistance training [335]. The decline in estrogen during menopause is thought to be one reason why muscle strength declines more in older women than in older men, in whom the decline is more linear [336]. Estrogen clearly appears to be important for muscle mass in women, as estrogen therapy positively affects muscle mass and strength in older women [337,338] while also increasing myofibrillar protein synthesis in response to resistance training [339]. Thus, estrogen appears to be anabolic when administered to older women undergoing resistance training and may attenuate muscle decline during aging.

RESISTANCE TRAINING DURING PREGNANCY

Pregnancy is associated with major physiological and psychological changes that often lead to lower levels of physical activity. According to observational studies, not even one-fifth of all pregnant women achieve the recommendation of 150 minutes of weekly physical activity at moderate intensity [340]. Reduced physical activity may contribute to an increased risk of gestational diabetes, hypertension, weight gain, and cardiovascular disease [341]. The literature suggests that most women maintain some weight gain after pregnancy, so physical activity, along with other lifestyle factors, may be important to control excessive weight gain during pregnancy.

Physical activity is generally considered safe for both the pregnant woman and the fetus. There is no increased risk of adverse pregnancy or birth outcomes. On the contrary, physical activity may help prevent some of the pregnancy complications mentioned above. Therefore, pregnant women should try to be physically active for at least 150 minutes per week and perform muscle-strengthening activities at least twice per week.

Even though physical activity is generally safe and beneficial for pregnant women, some caution is advised. Contact sports and activities where there is an obvious risk of falling should be avoided. In addition, pregnancy-related symptoms and complications should be managed in consultation with the physician and midwife.

There is relatively little information on the effects of resistance training during pregnancy. However, some of the physiological changes that occur during pregnancy may affect how resistance training can and should be performed. Hormonal changes lead to increased joint mobility, and overall weight gain causes bones, joints and muscles to be loaded differently during resistance training. The center of gravity also shifts forward, which can affect the performance of certain exercises and increase stress in the lumbar spine. In the supine position, venous return is prevented from about the fourth month of pregnancy, which is why women should avoid resistance training in the supine position after 16 weeks of pregnancy.

As the abdomen grows, the distance between the superficial abdominal muscles increases, which is called rectus diastasis. Together with the change in center of gravity, this can lead to decreased trunk stability. Pregnant women should also avoid maximal strains, which can trigger contraction reflexes. They should also be careful not to increase body temperature too much to protect against heat stress [342].

Pelvic floor exercises during pregnancy and after delivery can prevent and treat urine leakage [343]. Therefore, all women are recommended to perform such exercise. Intervention studies have shown that general muscle–strengthening programs are safe for pregnant women to perform and lead to increased strength [344]. There are still too few intervention studies to confidently assess whether resistance training leads to improved birth outcomes or health after pregnancy [345]. A combination of resistance and endurance training is often recommended during and after pregnancy, and there is strong evidence that such training is associated with overall improved fitness and prevention of urinary incontinence [345].

In summary, muscle–strengthening exercise in combination with specific pelvic floor exercises is recommended during pregnancy. Considering the reasonable precautions discussed in this section, a practical recommendation may be to perform resistance training 2–3 times per week in a controlled manner with moderate loads (>10 repetitions). Exercises in the supine position, exercises that place high demands on balance, and exercises that require breath holding and a great deal of pressure on the abdomen should be avoided.

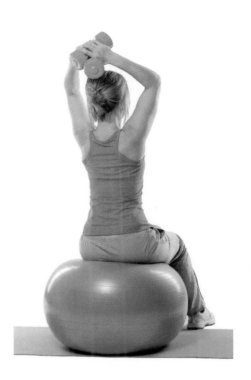

RESISTANCE TRAINING FOR ATHLETES

The underlying principles of resistance training physiology are equally valid for athletes and non–athletes. However, what distinguishes athletes from others is their specific approach to resistance training to improve their performance in a particular sport. Resistance training for adult athletes should therefore focus primarily on muscle groups and muscle actions that are relevant to the sport in question. This can be achieved, for example, by training force production during a particular sport–specific movement. The benefits of resistance training can also be indirect, for example, resistance training can reduce the risk of injury. The specific requirements of the sport should always be the starting point for the training plan. Important factors to consider may include:

- ✦ What joints are involved in the sport?
- ✦ What types of forceful actions are required?
- ✦ What movement patterns and contraction types are most common?
- ✦ What energy systems are active?
- ✦ What joint angles and movement patterns are common in this sport?
- ✦ What muscle groups and joints are most commonly injured?
- ✦ What body composition is beneficial?
- ✦ What physical skills are most important in the sport?

In a sports context, resistance training is often periodized based on an annual training schedule, which in turn is based on the distribution of competitions or games during a season. A regular annual plan often includes a preparation period, a competition period, and a transition period. Each period is divided into macrocycles, mesocycles, and microcycles, which define the physiological adaptations targeted during each phase. Another goal of periodization may be to ensure varied training, adequate recovery, or tapering before competition.

In sports that focus on only one or a few individual competitions per year, a linear periodization model is often used. Here, a higher volume of training is often followed by a period of lower volume but higher intensity and/or greater focus on sport–specific exercises as competition approaches. Shortly before important competitions, a tapering phase is usually carried out in which the training volume is greatly reduced.

For team athletes whose competitions are spread out over a large portion of the calendar year, resistance training is often prioritized in the preseason and then performed at maintenance levels during periods of frequent competition. A relatively small amount of resistance training is sufficient to maintain muscular strength and explosive power and can still prevent injury. Athletes should therefore avoid prolonged breaks from resistance training during the season. This would also reduce the need for recovery from muscle fatigue and exercise–induced muscle soreness, which often occur when heavy resistance training is performed less frequently.

Resistance training is central to sports where the ability to develop high forces is an important factor in performance. These include sports such as powerlifting, Olympic weightlifting, throwing disciplines, and wrestling. As mentioned in the chapter on concurrent training, resistance training can also improve sport–specific performance in endurance–oriented sports such as running, skiing, and cycling. These effects are achieved through a combination of different adaptations that are beneficial for endurance athletes, such as improved running economy, increased power output at the end of a race, or a better ability to maintain a higher pace in the fatigued state.

In team sports, resistance training can be an adjunct to sport–specific exercises and allow for high loads in specific actions where it is difficult to achieve overloads in certain parts of a movement. Resistance training can thus contribute to increased speed and/or power development during sport–specific actions such as sprints, changes of direction, tackles, and jumps.

In addition to sport–specific needs, resistance training in general can be used by athletes who want to change their body composition or reduce the overall risk of muscle injury. To change body composition, high protein intake and reduced calorie intake should accompany resistance training to maintain or increase muscle mass while reducing fat mass.

To reduce the risk of injury, a combination of different types of exercises and loads is often used. Some simple exercises for the hamstring and adductor muscles, for example, have been shown to reduce the risk of muscle injury in team sports, while stability and balance exercises can reduce the risk of knee and ankle injuries. A poorly rehabilitated injury often leads to new injuries, and the number of injuries is in turn closely related to performance in both individual and team sports. The use of resistance training as a means of reducing the risk of injury is therefore important in virtually all sports.

SPOTLIGHT
Can you increase your strength without gaining muscle?
· ·

In many sports where one's body weight must be supported, it is desirable to increase muscular strength and explosiveness without increasing body weight or building "unnecessary" muscle mass. Athletes pursuing this goal should favor resistance training with high loads and explosive movement execution. With such training, the total training volume can be kept low, and neural and extracellular matrix adaptations are stimulated to a greater extent than muscle growth. In addition, it is important to perform the exercise according to the principle of specificity to ensure that the increased strength contributes to sport–specific performance. To achieve the maximum transfer effect of resistance training to a complex sport, it is essential to combine different types of resistance training that include both heavy and lighter loads, basic and specific exercises, and different types of jumps, accelerations and changes of direction [346].

SUMMARY

➲ The age–related loss of muscle mass and strength is called sarcopenia.

➲ Muscle mass begins to decrease in the 30s to 40s, and after the 60–70s the loss continues to increase.

➲ The cause of sarcopenia is multifactorial, with important contributing factors being neuromuscular degeneration, changes in protein turnover and satellite cell function, changes in hormone levels, chronic inflammation and oxidative stress, and lifestyle factors such as physical inactivity and unhealthy diet.

➲ Resistance training is generally safe for children and adolescents. Emphasis should be placed on exercises perceived as fun, motivating, and challenging.

➲ The risks of resistance training for children are mainly related to accidents, excessive loading, or improper technique.

➲ Properly performed resistance training in adolescence can be a good addition to the general training schedule and helps improve motor skills, increase strength, and reduce the risk of injury.

➲ Both women and men respond well to resistance training when it comes to increasing muscle mass and strength.

➲ Although men are stronger and have more muscle mass than women, sex differences in response to exercise are small, if they exist at all.

➲ The most obvious difference between men and women is the difference in levels of the sex hormones testosterone and estrogen. However, these differences in hormone production do not appear to have a major impact on muscle protein turnover at rest or after resistance training.

➲ During pregnancy, there are major physiological and psychological changes that often result in reduced physical activity.

➲ Physical activity can help prevent pregnancy complications. All pregnant women are recommended to engage in at least 150 minutes of physical activity per week and to perform muscle–strengthening exercises at least twice a week, as well as specific pelvic floor exercises to prevent urine leakage.

➲ The hormonal changes during pregnancy cause increased joint mobility, and the overall weight gain causes bones, joints, and muscles to be loaded differently during resistance training while also shifting the center of gravity.

➲ Pregnant women should avoid maximum loads that can trigger sudden contraction reflexes, avoid supine resistance training after 16 weeks of pregnancy, avoid contact sports and the risk of falling, and be careful not to increase body temperature too much.

➲ Athletes should plan resistance training based on the profile of the sport and the distribution of competitions and games during the season.

➲ Resistance training is capable of increasing performance in sport–specific actions and reducing the risk of injury.

➲ Many athletes want to increase their strength without gaining muscle mass. To achieve this, resistance training should be performed using a combination of heavier and lighter loads that increase maximal and explosive strength, while keeping the overall training load low to avoid significant muscle hypertrophy.

➲ To achieve the maximum transfer effect of resistance training to a complex sport, it is important to combine different types of resistance training that include heavy and lighter loads, basic and specific exercises, as well as different types of jumps, accelerations, and changes of direction.

FIGURE REFERENCES

Figure 1.1.   The image was reworked from an original image created by OpenStax. The image was released under the Creative Commons Attribution 4.0 International license (https://creativecommons. org/licenses/by/4.0/deed.en), which allows the image to be reworked and distributed if the original source is credited. Image downloaded from https://commons.wikimedia.org/wiki/ File:1007_Muscle_Fibes_(large).jpg

Figure 1.2.   The image was reworked from an original image created by BruceBlaus. The image was released under the Creative Commons Attribution–Share Alike 4.0 International license (https://creativecommons.org/licenses/by–sa/4.0/), which allows editing and distribution of the image if the original source is credited and the image is published under the same terms as the original image. The image was downloaded from https://commons.wikimedia.org/wiki/ File:Muscle_Types.png.

Figure 1.3.   The image was reworked based on an original image created by OpenStax. The image was released under the Creative Commons Attribution 4.0 International license (https:// creativecommons.org/licenses/by/4.0/deed.en), which allows the image to be reworked and distributed if the original source is credited. The image was downloaded from https://upload. wikimedia.org/wikipedia/commons/9/9c/1022_Muscle_Fibers_%28small%29.jpg.

Figure 2.4.   The image was reworked from an original image created by Dhp1080. The image was released under the Creative Commons Attribution–Share Alike 3.0 International license (https:// creativecommons.org/licenses/by–sa/3.0/), which allows editing and distribution of the image if the original source is credited and the image is published under the same terms as the original image. The image was downloaded from https://upload.wikimedia.org/wikipedia/commons/ thumb/b/b5/Neuron.svg/1280px–Neuron.svg.png.

Figure 2.8.   The image was reworked based on an original image created by OpenStax. The image was released under the Creative Commons Attribution 4.0 International license ((https:// creativecommons.org/licenses/by/4.0/deed.en), which allows the image to be revised and distributed if the original source is credited. The image was downloaded from https: // commons.wikimedia.org/wiki/File:1010a_Contraction_new.jpg

Figure 3.2. The image was reworked from an original image created by OpenStax. The image was released under the Creative Commons Attribution 4.0 International license, which allows reworking and distribution of the image if the original source is credited. The image was downloaded from https://commons.wikimedia.org/wiki/File:1015_Types_of_Contraction_new.jpg.

Figure 4.1. Figure based on data from Phillips SM, Tipton KD, Aarsland A, Wolf SE, Wolfe RR. Mixed muscle protein synthesis and breakdown after resistance exercise in humans. Am J Physiol. 1997, 273 (1): E 99–107.

Figure 4.2. Figure based on data from Tang JE, Perco JG, Moore DR, Wilkinson SB, Phillips SM. Resistance training alters the response of fed state mixed muscle protein synthesis in young men. Am J Physiol Regul Integr Comp Physiol. 2008. 294(1): R172–8.

Figure 5.1. Figure based on data from Narici MV, Hoppeler H, Kayser B, Landoni L, Claassen H, Gavardi C, Conti M, Cerretelli P. Human quadriceps cross–sectional area, torque and neural activation during 6 months resistance training. Acta Physiol Scand. 1996.157 (2): 175–86.

Figure 6.2. Figure based on data from Lundberg TR, García–Gutiérrez MT, Mandic M, Lilja M, Fernandez–Gonzalo R. Regional and muscle–specific adaptations in knee extensor hypertrophy using flywheel vs. conventional weight–stack resistance exercise. Appl Physiol Nutr Metab. 2019, 44(8):827–833.

Figure 6.3. Figure based on data from Lundberg TR, Fernandez–Gonzalo R, Gustafsson T, Tesch PA. Aerobic exercise does not compromise muscle hypertrophy response to short–term resistance training. J Appl Physiol. 2013, 1; 114 (1): 81–9.

Figure 6.4. Figure based on data from Lundberg TR, Fernandez–Gonzalo R, Gustafsson T, Tesch PA. Aerobic exercise does not compromise muscle hypertrophy response to short–term resistance training. J Appl Physiol. 2013, 1; 114 (1): 81–9.

Figure 7.1. Figure is redrawn from a figure in Egan B, Zierath JR. Exercise metabolism and the molecular regulation of skeletal muscle adaptation. Cell Metab. 2013, 5; 17 (2): 162–84 .

Figure 9.2. Figure based on data from Seynnes OR, The Boer M, Narici MV. Early skeletal muscle hypertrophy and architectural changes in response to high–intensity resistance training. J Appl Physiol. 2007, 102 (1): 368–73.

Figure 11.1. Figure based on data from Morton RW, Murphy KT, McKellar SR, Schoenfeld BJ, Henselmans M, Helms E, Aragon AA, Devries MC, Banfield L, Krieger JW, Phillips SM. A systematic review, meta–analysis and meta–regression of the effect of protein supplementation on resistance training in muscle mass and strength in healthy adults. Br J Sports Med. 2018, 52 (6): 376–384.

Figure 15.1. Figure based on data from Hickson RC. Interference of strength development by simultaneously training for strength and endurance. Eur J Appl Physiol Occup Physiol. 1980; 45 (2–3): 255–63.

REFERENCES

1. Kraemer WJ, Häkkinen K. Strength Training for Sport. Blackwell Science; 2002.

2. Kraemer WJ et al. Understanding the Science of Resistance Training: An Evolutionary Perspective. Sports Med; 2017.

3. Svett & korsett: Mediko–mekaniskt gym; 2016.

4. Holmes JW. Teaching from classic papers: Hill's model of muscle contraction. Adv Physiol Educ; 2006.

5. Huxley AF. The origin of force in skeletal muscle. Ciba Found Symp; 1975.

6. Nuzzo JL. History of Strength Training Research in Man: An Inventory and Quantitative Overview of Studies Published in English Between 1894 and 1979. J Strength Cond Res; 2021.

7. Delorme TL, Watkins AL. Technics of progressive resistance exercise. Arch Phys Med Rehabil; 1948.

8. Berger R. Effect of Varied Weight Training Programs on Strength. Res Q Am Assoc Health Phys Educ Recreat; 1962.

9. Müller E. Training Muscle Strength. Ergonomics; 1959.

10. Henneman E. Relation between size of neurons and their susceptibility to discharge. Science; 1957.

11. Moritani T, deVries H. Neural factors versus hypertrophy in the time course of muscle strength gain. Am J Phys Med; 1979.

12. Narici MV et al. Muscle structural assembly and functional consequences. J Exp Biol; 2016.

13. Olsson K et al. Intracellular Ca^{2+}–handling differs markedly between intact human muscle fibers and myotubes. Skelet Muscle; 2015.

14. Hoppeler H et al. The ultrastructure of the normal human skeletal muscle. A morphometric analysis on untrained men, women and well–trained orienteers. Pflugers Arch; 1973.

15. Nuzzo JL. Sex differences in skeletal muscle fiber types: A meta–analysis. Clin Anat; 2023.

16. Sale D. Neural adaptations to strength training. In: Strength and Power in Sport. Blackwell Science; 2003.

17. Franchi MV et al. Skeletal muscle remodeling in response to eccentric vs. concentric loading: Morphological, molecular, and metabolic adaptations. Front Physiol; 2017.

18. Hessel AL et al. Physiological mechanisms of eccentric contraction and its applications: A role for the giant titin protein. Front Physiol; 2017.

19. Ramaswamy KS et al. Lateral transmission of force is impaired in skeletal muscles of dystrophic mice and very old rats. J Physiol; 2011.

20. Maruyama K. Connectin, an elastic protein from myofibrils. J Biochem Tokyo; 1976.

21. Herzog W. The multiple roles of titin in muscle contraction and force production. Biophys Rev; 2018.

22. Stokes T et al. Recent perspectives regarding the role of dietary protein for the promotion of muscle hypertrophy with resistance exercise training. Nutrients; 2018.

23. Smeets JSJ et al. Brain tissue plasticity: Protein synthesis rates of the human brain. Brain; 2018.

24. Wilkinson SB et al. Differential effects of resistance and endurance exercise in the fed state on signalling molecule phosphorylation and protein synthesis in human muscle. J Physiol; 2008.

25. Wilkinson DJ et al. A validation of the application of D(2)O stable isotope tracer techniques for monitoring day–to–day changes in muscle protein subfraction synthesis in humans. Am J Physiol Endocrinol Metab; 2014.

26. Greenhaff PL et al. Disassociation between the effects of amino acids and insulin on signaling, ubiquitin ligases, and protein turnover in human muscle. Am J Physiol Endocrinol Metab; 2008.

27. Damas F et al. A Review of Resistance Training–Induced Changes in Skeletal Muscle Protein Synthesis and Their Contribution to Hypertrophy. Sports Med; 2015.

28. Damas F et al. Muscle protein synthesis, hypertrophy, and muscle damage in humans. J Physiol; 2017.

29. Kumar V et al. Human muscle protein synthesis and breakdown during and after exercise. J Appl Physiol; 2009.

30. Mitchell CJ et al. Acute post–exercise myofibrillar protein synthesis is not correlated with resistance training–induced muscle hypertrophy in young men. PLoS One; 2014.

31. Damas F et al. Early resistance training–induced increases in muscle cross–sectional area are concomitant with edema–induced muscle swelling. Eur J Appl Physiol; 2016.

32. Hubal MJ et al. Muscle Size and Strength Gain after Unilateral Resistance Training. Med Sci Sports Exerc; 2005.

33. Narici MV et al. Human quadriceps cross–sectional area, torque and neural activation during 6 months strength training. Acta Physiol Scand; 1996.

34. Van Cutsem M et al. Changes in single motor unit behaviour contribute to the increase in contraction speed after dynamic training in humans. J Physiol; 1998.

35. Siddique U et al. Determining the Sites of Neural Adaptations to Resistance Training: A Systematic Review and Meta–analysis. Sports Med; 2020.

36. Miller RG et al. Rate of tension development in isometric contractions of a human hand muscle. Exp Neurol; 1981.

37. Folland JP, Williams AG. The adaptations to strength training: Morphological and neurological contributions to increased strength. Sports Med; 2007.

38. Häkkinen K, Komi PV, Alen M. Effect of explosive type strength training on isometric force– and relaxation–time, electromyographic and muscle fibre characteristics of leg extensor muscles. Acta Physiol Scand; 1985.

39. Häkkinen K, Alen M, Komi PV. Changes in isometric force– and relaxation–time, electromyographic and muscle fibre characteristics of human skeletal muscle during strength training and detraining. Acta Physiol Scand; 1985.

40. de Luca CJ et al. Behaviour of human motor units in different muscles during linearly varying contractions. J Physiol; 1982.

41. Duchateau J, Semmler JG, Enoka RM. Training adaptations in the behavior of human motor units. J Appl Physiol Bethesda Md; 2006.

42. Del Vecchio A et al. The increase in muscle force after 4 weeks of strength training is mediated by adaptations in motor unit recruitment and rate coding. J Physiol; 2019.

43. Dideriksen JL, Del Vecchio A, Farina D. Neural and muscular determinants of maximal rate of force development. J Neurophysiol; 2020.

44. Balshaw TG et al. Reduced firing rates of high threshold motor units in response to eccentric overload. Physiol Rep; 2017.

45. Behm DG et al. Intermuscle differences in activation. Muscle Nerve; 2002.

46. Balshaw TG et al. Neural adaptations after 4 years vs. 12 weeks of resistance training vs. untrained. Scand J Med Sci Sports; 2018.

47. Gabriel DA et al. Neural adaptations to resistive exercise: mechanisms and recommendations for training practices. Sports Med; 2006.

48. Suchomel TJ et al. The Importance of Muscular Strength: Training Considerations. Sports Med; 2018.

49. Amiridis IG et al. Co–activation and tension regulating phenomena during isokinetic knee extension in sedentary and highly skilled humans. Eur J Appl Physiol; 1996.

50. Westing SH et al. Effects of electrical stimulation on eccentric and concentric torque–velocity relationships during knee extension in man. Acta Physiol Scand; 1990.

51. Aagaard P et al. Neural inhibition during maximal eccentric and concentric quadriceps contraction: effects of resistance training. J Appl Physiol; 2000.

52. Aagaard P et al. Increased rate of force development and neural drive of human skeletal muscle following resistance training. J Appl Physiol; 2002.

53. Robbins DW. Postactivation potentiation and its practical applicability: A brief review. J Strength Cond Res; 2005.

54. Tillin NA, Bishop D. Factors modulating post–activation potentiation and its effect on performance of subsequent explosive activities. Sports Med; 2009.

55. Haun CT et al. A Critical Evaluation of the Biological Construct Skeletal Muscle Hypertrophy: Size Matters but So Does the Measurement. Front Physiol; 2019.

56. Roberts MD et al. Mechanisms of mechanical overload–induced skeletal muscle hypertrophy: current understanding and future directions. Physiol Rev; 2023.

57. Karlsson A et al. Automatic and quantitative assessment of regional muscle volume by multi–atlas segmentation using whole–body water–fat MRI. J Magn Reson Imaging; 2015.

58. Alway SE et al. Effects of strength training and immobilization on human muscle fibres. Eur J Appl Physiol Occup Physiol; 1992.

59. Radaelli R et al. Time course of low– and high–volume strength training on neuromuscular adaptations and muscle quality in older women. Age; 2014.

60. Wernbom M et al. The influence of frequency, intensity, volume and mode of strength training on whole muscle cross–sectional area in humans. Sports Med; 2007.

61. Lundberg TR et al. Aerobic exercise does not compromise muscle hypertrophy response to short–term resistance training. J Appl Physiol; 2013.

62. Illera–Domínguez V et al. Early functional and morphological muscle adaptations during short–term inertial–squat training. Front Physiol; 2018.

63. Tesch PA, Larsson L. Muscle hypertrophy in bodybuilders. Eur J Appl Physiol Occup Physiol; 1982.

64.   Eriksson A et al. Hypertrophic muscle fibers with fissures in power–lifters; fiber splitting or defect regeneration? Histochem Cell Biol; 2006.

65.   Schantz P. Capillary supply in hypertrophied human skeletal muscle. Acta Physiol Scand; 1982.

66.   Gollnick PD et al. Muscular enlargement and number of fibers in skeletal muscles of rats. J Appl Physiol; 1981.

67.   Kelley G. Mechanical overload and skeletal muscle fiber hyperplasia: a meta–analysis. J Appl Physiol; 1996.

68.   Murach KA et al. Muscle Fiber Splitting is a Physiological Response to Extreme Loading in Animals. Exerc Sport Sci Rev; 2019.

69.   Sjöström M et al. Evidence of fibre hyperplasia in human skeletal muscles from healthy young men? – A left–right comparison of the fibre number in whole anterior tibialis muscles. Eur J Appl Physiol; 1991.

70.   MacDougall JD et al. Effects of strength training and immobilization on human muscle fibres. Eur J Appl Physiol Occup Physiol; 1980.

71.   Roberts MD et al. Sarcoplasmic Hypertrophy in Skeletal Muscle: A Scientific 'Unicorn' or Resistance Training Adaptation? Front Physiol; 2020.

72.   Haun CT et al. Muscle fiber hypertrophy in response to 6 weeks of high–volume resistance training in trained young men is largely attributed to sarcoplasmic hypertrophy. PLoSOne; 2019.

73.   Jorgenson KW et al. Identifying the Structural Adaptations that Drive the Mechanical Load–Induced Growth of Skeletal Muscle: A Scoping Review. Cells; 2020.

74.   Horwath O et al. Variability in vastus lateralis fiber type distribution, fiber size, and myonuclear content along and between the legs. J Appl Physiol; 2021.

75.   Morkin E. Postnatal muscle fiber assembly: Localization of newly synthesized myofibrillar proteins. Science; 1970.

76.   Andersen LL. Changes in the human muscle force–velocity relationship in response to resistance training and subsequent detraining. J Appl Physiol; 2005.

77.   Tobias IS, Galpin AJ. Moving human muscle physiology research forward: an evaluation of fiber type-specific protein research methodologies. Am J Physiol Cell Physiol; 2020.

78.   Wilmore JH. Alterations in strength, body composition and anthropometric measurements consequent to a 10–week weight training program. Med Sci Sports; 1974.

79.   Cureton KJ et al. Hypertrophy in Men and Women.pdf. Med Sci Sports Exerc; 1988.

80.   Welle S et al. Effect of age on muscle hypertrophy induced by resistance training. J Gerontol Ser Biol Sci Med Sci; 1996.

81.   Gejl KD et al. Contractile Properties of MHC I and II Fibers From Highly Trained Arm and Leg Muscles of Cross-Country Skiers. Front Physiol; 2021.

82.   Fiatarone MA et al. High–Intensity Strength Training in Nonagenarians: Effects on Skeletal Muscle. JAMA J Am Med Assoc; 1990.

83.   Greig CA et al. Blunting of adaptive responses to resistance exercise training in women over 75y. Exp Gerontol; 2011.

84.   Suetta C et al. Effects of aging on human skeletal muscle after immobilization and retraining. J Appl Physiol; 2009.

85.   Cotofana S et al. Correlation between single–slice muscle anatomical cross–sectional area and muscle volume in thigh extensors, flexors and adductors of perimenopausal women. Eur J Appl Physiol; 2010.

86. Churchward–Venne TA et al. There are no nonresponders to resistance–type exercise training inolder men and women. J Am Med Dir Assoc; 2015.

87. Roberts MD et al. Physiological differences between low versus high skeletal muscle hypertrophic responders to resistance exercise training: Current perspectives and future research directions. Front Physiol; 2018.

88. Timmons JA. Variability in training–induced skeletal muscle adaptation. J Appl Physiol; 2011.

89. Buckner SL et al. The problem of muscle hypertrophy: Revisited. Muscle Nerve; 2016.

90. Wackerhage H et al. Stimuli and sensors that initiate skeletal muscle hypertrophy following resistance exercise. J Appl Physiol; 2018.

91. Fowles JR et al. The Effects of Acute Passive Stretch on Muscle Protein Synthesis in Humans. Can J Appl Physiol; 2000.

92. Mounier R et al. Expanding roles for AMPK in skeletal muscle plasticity. Trends Endocrinol Metab; 2015.

93. Dunn SE et al. Calcineurin is required for skeletal muscle hypertrophy. J Biol Chem; 1999.

94. Scheele C et al. ROS and myokines promote muscle adaptation to exercise. Trends Endocrinol Metab; 2009.

95. Millar ID et al. Mammary protein synthesis is acutely regulated by the cellular hydration state. Biochem Biophys Res Commun; 1997.

96. Dangott B et al. Dietary creatine monohydrate supplementation increases satellite cell mitotic activity during compensatory hypertrophy. Int J Sports Med; 2000.

97. Hartgens F, Kuipers H. Effects of androgenic–anabolic steroids in athletes. Sports Med; 2004.

98. Sinha–Hikim I et al. Testosterone–induced muscle hypertrophy is associated with an increase in satellite cell number in healthy, young men. Am J Physiol Endocrinol Metab; 2003.

99. Hickson RC et al. Skeletal muscle cytosol [3H]methyltrienolone receptor binding and serum androgens: Effects of hypertrophy and hormonal state. J Steroid Biochem; 1983.

100. Kvorning T et al. Suppression of endogenous testosterone production attenuates the response to strength training: a randomized, placebo–controlled, and blinded intervention study. Am J Physiol Endocrinol Metab; 2006.

101. Roberts BM, Nuckols G, Krieger JW. Sex Differences in Resistance Training: A Systematic Review and Meta–Analysis. J Strength Cond Res; 2020.

102. West DWD et al. Elevations in ostensibly anabolic hormones with resistance exercise enhance neither training–induced muscle hypertrophy nor strength of the elbow flexors. J Appl Physiol; 2010.

103. Spangenburg EE, Le Roith D, Ward CW, Bodine SC. A functional insulin–like growth factor receptor is not necessary for load–induced skeletal muscle hypertrophy. J Physiol; 2008.

104. Snijders T, Parise G. Role of muscle stem cells in sarcopenia. Curr Opin Clin Nutr Metab Care; 2017.

105. Sexton CL et al. Skeletal Muscle DNA Methylation and mRNA Responses to a Bout of Higher versus Lower Load Resistance Exercise in Previously Trained Men. Cells; 2023.

106. Goldberg AL, Egg J, Goldspink DF, Jablecki C. Mechanism of work–induced hypertrophy of skeletal muscle. Med Sci Sports; 1975.

107. Raue U et al. Transcriptome signature of resistance exercise adaptations: mixed muscle and fiber type specific profiles in young and old adults. J Appl Physiol; 2012.

108. Schuelke M et al. Myostatin mutation associated with gross muscle hypertrophy in a child. N Engl J Med; 2004.

109. Cunha TF et al. Aerobic exercise training upregulates skeletal muscle calpain and ubiquitin–proteasome systems in healthy mice. J Appl Physiol; 2012.

110. Hwee DT, Baehr LM, Philp A, Baar K, Bodine SC. Maintenance of muscle mass and load–induced growth in Muscle RING Finger 1 null mice with age. Aging Cell; 2014.

111. Hitachi K, Tsuchida K. Role of microRNAs in skeletal muscle hypertrophy. Front Physiol; 2014.

112. Kirby TJ, McCarthy JJ. MicroRNAs in skeletal muscle biology and exercise adaptation. Free Radic Biol Med; 2013.

113. Wong TS, Booth FW. Protein metabolism in rat gastrocnemius muscle after stimulated chronic concentric exercise. J Appl Physiol; 1990.

114. Bodine SC et al. Akt/mTOR pathway is a crucial regulator of skeletal muscle hypertrophy and can prevent muscle atrophy in vivo. Nat Cell Biol; 2001.

115. Baar K, Esser K. Phosphorylation of p70 S6k correlates with increased skeletal muscle mass following resistance exercise. Am J Physiol Cell Physiol; 1999.

116. Terzis G et al. Resistance exercise–induced increase in muscle mass correlates with p70S6 kinase phosphorylation in human subjects. Eur J Appl Physiol; 2008.

117. Mayhew DL et al. Translational signaling responses preceding resistance training–mediated myofiber hypertrophy in young and old humans. J Appl Physiol; 2009.

118. von Walden F. Ribosome biogenesis in skeletal muscle: coordination of transcription and translation. J Appl Physiol Bethesda Md; 2019.

119. Murach KA et al. Differential requirement for satellite cells during overload–induced muscle hypertrophy in growing versus mature mice. Skelet Muscle; 2017.

120. Jackson JR et al. Satellite cell depletion does not inhibit adult skeletal muscle regrowth following unloading–induced atrophy. Am J Physiol Cell Physiol; 2012.

121. Petrella JK et al. Efficacy of myonuclear addition may explain differential myofiber growth among resistance–trained young and older men and women. Am J Physiol Endocrinol Metab; 2006.

122. Conceicao MS et al. Muscle Fiber Hypertrophy and Myonuclei Addition: A Systematic Review and Meta–analysis. Med Sci Sports Exerc; 2018.

123. Staron RS et al. Strength and skeletal muscle adaptations in heavy–resistance–trained women after detraining and retraining. J Appl Physiol; 1991.

124. Kadi F, Eriksson A, Holmner S, Thornell LE. Effects of anabolic steroids on the muscle cells of strength–trained athletes. Med Sci Sports Exerc; 1999.

125. Nielsen JL et al. Higher myonuclei density in muscle fibers persists among former users of anabolic androgenic steroids. J Clin Endocrinol Metab; 2023.

126. Murach KA et al. 'Muscle Memory' Not Mediated By Myonuclear Number?: Secondary Analysis of Human Detraining Data. J Appl Physiol; 2019.

127. Rahmati M, McCarthy JJ, Malakoutinia F. Myonuclear permanence in skeletal muscle memory: a systematic review and meta–analysis of human and animal studies. J Cachexia Sarcopenia Muscle; 2022.

128. Seaborne RA et al. Human Skeletal Muscle Possesses an Epigenetic Memory of Hypertrophy. Sci Rep; 2018.

129. Lindholm ME et al. The Impact of Endurance Training on Human Skeletal Muscle Memory, Global Isoform Expression and Novel Transcripts. PLoS Genet; 2016.

130. Tipton KD, Hamilton DL, Gallagher IJ. Assessing the Role of Muscle Protein Breakdown in Response to Nutrition and Exercise in Humans. Sports Med; 2018.

131. Dudley GA, Tesch PA, Harris RT, Golden CL, Buchanan P. Influence of eccentric actions on the metabolic cost of resistance exercise. Aviat Space Environ Med; 1991.

132. Cunha FA et al. Concurrent exercise circuit protocol performed in public fitness facilities meets the ACSM guidelines for energy cost and metabolic intensity among older adults in Rio de Janeiro City. Appl Physiol Nutr Metab Physiol Appl Nutr Metab; 2018.

133. Tesch P, Alkner B. Acute and Chronic Muscle Metabolic Adaptations to Strength Training. In: Strength and Power in Sport. Blackwell Science; 2003.

134. Tesch PA, Colliander EB, Kaiser P. Muscle metabolism during intense, heavy-resistance exercise. Eur J Appl Physiol; 1986.

135. Verdijk LB et al. Resistance Training Increases Skeletal Muscle Capillarization in Healthy Older Men. Med Sci Sports Exerc; 2016.

136. Holloway TM et al. Temporal Response of Angiogenesis and Hypertrophy to Resistance Training in Young Men. Med Sci Sports Exerc; 2018.

137. Nederveen JP et al. The influence of capillarization on satellite cell pool expansion and activation following exercise-induced muscle damage in healthy young men. J Physiol; 2018.

138. Nederveen JP et al. Skeletal muscle satellite cells are located at a closer proximity to capillaries in healthy young compared with older men. J Cachexia Sarcopenia Muscle; 2016.

139. Snijders T et al. Muscle fibre capillarization is a critical factor in muscle fibre hypertrophy during resistance exercise training in older men. J Cachexia Sarcopenia Muscle; 2017.

140. Lundberg TR et al. Early accentuated muscle hypertrophy is strongly associated with myonuclear accretion. Am J Physiol Regul Integr Comp Physiol; 2020.

141. Tang JE, Hartman JW, Phillips SM. Increased muscle oxidative potential following resistance training induced fibre hypertrophy in young men. Appl Physiol Nutr Metab; 2006.

142. Porter C et al. Resistance Exercise Training Alters Mitochondrial Function in Human Skeletal Muscle. Med Sci Sports Exerc; 2015.

143. Cardinale DA et al. Resistance Training with Co-ingestion of Anti-inflammatory Drugs Attenuates Mitochondrial Function. Front Physiol; 2017.

144. Trommelen J et al. Exogenous insulin does not increase muscle protein synthesis rate when administered systemically: A systematic review. Eur J Endocrinol; 2015.

145. DeVol DL et al. Activation of insulin-like growth factor gene expression during work-induced skeletal muscle growth. Am J Physiol Endocrinol Metab; 1990.

146. Mitchell CJ et al. Muscular and systemic correlates of resistance training-induced muscle hypertrophy. PLoS One; 2013.

147. Bhasin S et al. The effects of supraphysiologic doses of testosterone on muscle size and strength in normal men. N Engl J Med; 1996.

148. Handelsman DJ, Hirschberg AL, Bermon S. Circulating testosterone as the hormonal basis of sex differences in athletic performance. Endocr Rev; 2018.

149. Hoffmann C, Weigert C. Skeletal muscle as an endocrine organ: The role of myokines in exercise adaptations. Cold Spring Harb Perspect Med; 2017.

150. Trappe TA et al. Influence of acetaminophen and ibuprofen on skeletal muscle adaptations to resistance exercise in older adults. Am J Physiol Regul Integr Comp Physiol; 2011.

151. Lieber RL. Can we just forget about pennation angle? J Biomech; 2022.

152. Aagaard P et al. A mechanism for increased contractile strength of human pennate muscle in response to strength training: Changes in muscle architecture. J Physiol; 2001.

153. Seynnes OR et al. Early skeletal muscle hypertrophy and architectural changes in response to high-intensity resistance training. J Appl Physiol; 2007.

154. Franchi MV et al. Architectural, functional and molecular responses to concentric and eccentric loading in human skeletal muscle. Acta Physiol; 2014.

155. Jorgenson KW, Hornberger TA. The Overlooked Role of Fiber Length in Mechanical Load–Induced Growth of Skeletal Muscle. Exerc Sport Sci Rev; 2019.

156. Magnusson SP, Kjaer M. The impact of loading, unloading, ageing and injury on the human tendon. J Physiol; 2018.

157. Heinemeier KM et al. Lack of tissue renewal in human adult Achilles tendon is revealed by nuclear bomb14C. FASEB J; 2013.

158. Hughes DC et al. Effects of aging, exercise, and disease on force transfer in skeletal muscle. Am J Physiol Endocrinol Metab; 2015.

159. MacDougall JD et al. Muscle fiber number in biceps brachii in bodybuilders and control subjects. J Appl Physiol; 1984.

160. Kosek DJ, Bamman MM. Modulation of the dystrophin–associated protein complex in response to resistance training in young and older men. J Appl Physiol; 2008.

161. Miller BF et al. Coordinated collagen and muscle protein synthesis in human patella tendon and quadriceps muscle after exercise. J Physiol; 2005.

162. Bohm S et al. Human tendon adaptation in response to mechanical loading: a systematic review and meta–analysis of exercise intervention studies on healthy adults. Sports Med Open; 2015.

163. Baar K. Minimizing Injury and Maximizing Return to Play: Lessons from Engineered Ligaments. Sports Med; 2017.

164. Ma D, Wu L, He Z. Effects of walking on the preservation of bone mineral density in perimenopausal and postmenopausal women: a systematic review and meta–analysis. Menopause; 2013.

165. Hong AR, Kim SW. Effects of Resistance Exercise on Bone Health. Endocrinol Metab Seoul Korea; 2018.

166. Klein–Nulend J et al. Mechanosensation and transduction in osteocytes. Bone; 2013.

167. Robling AG et al. Recovery periods restore mechanosensitivity to dynamically loaded bone. J Exp Biol; 2001.

168. Robling AG et al. Shorter, more frequent mechanical loading sessions enhance bone mass. Med Sci Sports Exerc; 2002.

169. Hortobágyi T et al. The effects of detraining on power athletes. Med Sci Sports Exerc; 1993.

170. Morrissey MC et al. Resistance training modes: specificity and effectiveness. Med Sci Sports Exerc; 1995.

171. Burd NA et al. Resistance exercise volume affects myofibrillar protein synthesis and anabolic signalling molecule phosphorylation in young men. J Physiol; 2010.

172. Schoenfeld BJ, Ogborn D, Krieger JW. Dose–response relationship between weekly resistance training volume and increases in muscle mass: A systematic review and meta–analysis. J Sports Sci; 2017.

173. Schoenfeld BJ et al. Resistance Training Volume Enhances Muscle Hypertrophy. Med Sci Sports Exerc; 2018.

174. Spiering BA et al. Are Trainees Lifting Heavy Enough? Self–Selected Loads in Resistance Exercise: A Scoping Review and Exploratory Meta–analysis. Sports Med; 2023.

175. Hammarström D et al. Benefits of higher resistance–training volume are related to ribosome biogenesis. J Physiol; 2020.

176. Grgic J, Schoenfeld BJ, Latella C. Resistance training frequency and skeletal muscle hypertrophy: A review of available evidence. Journal of Science and Medicine in Sport; 2018.

177. Schoenfeld BJ, Ogborn D, Krieger JW. Effects of Resistance Training Frequency on Measures of Muscle Hypertrophy: A Systematic Review and Meta–Analysis. Sports Med; 2016.

178. Grgic J et al. Effect of Resistance Training Frequency on Gains in Muscular Strength: A Systematic Review and Meta–Analysis. Sports Med; 2018.

179. Barcelos C et al. High–frequency resistance training does not promote greater muscular adaptations compared to low frequencies in young untrained men. Eur J Sport Sci; 2018.

180. Hamarsland H et al. Equal–Volume Strength Training With Different Training Frequencies Induces Similar Muscle Hypertrophy and Strength Improvement in Trained Participants. Front Physiol; 2021.

181. Henselmans M, Schoenfeld BJ. The effect of inter–set rest intervals on resistance exercise–induced muscle hypertrophy. Sports Med; 2014.

182. Schoenfeld BJ et al. Longer interset rest periods enhance muscle strength and hypertrophy in resistance–trained men. J Strength Cond Res; 2016.

183. McKendry J et al. Short inter–set rest blunts resistance exercise–induced increases in myofibrillar protein synthesis and intracellular signalling in young males. Exp Physiol; 2016.

184. Walker S et al. Neuromuscular fatigue in young and older men using constant or variable resistance. Eur J Appl Physiol; 2013.

185. Schoenfeld BJ. The mechanisms of muscle hypertrophy and their application to resistance training. J Strength Cond Res; 2010.

186. Bawa P et al. Rotation of motor neurons during prolonged isometric contractions in humans. J Neurophysiol; 2006.

187. Burd NA et al. Low–load high volume resistance exercise stimulates muscle protein synthesis more than high–load low volume resistance exercise in young men. PLoS One; 2010.

188. Mitchell CJ et al. Resistance exercise load does not determine training–mediated hypertrophic gains in young men. J Appl Physiol; 2012.

189. Morton RW et al. Neither load nor systemic hormones determine resistance training–mediated hypertrophy or strength gains in resistance–trained young men. J Appl Physiol; 2016.

190. Lasevicius T et al. Effects of different intensities of resistance training with equated volume load on muscle strength and hypertrophy. Eur J Sport Sci; 2018.

191. Steele J et al. Are Trainees Lifting Heavy Enough? Self–Selected Loads in Resistance Exercise: A Scoping Review and Exploratory Meta–analysis. Sports Med; 2022.

192. Schoenfeld BJ, Grgic J, Ogborn D, Krieger JW. Strength and hypertrophy adaptations between low– versus high–load resistance training. J Strength Cond Res; 2017.

193. Nóbrega SR et al. Effect of Resistance Training to Muscle Failure vs. Volitional Interruption at High– and Low–Intensities on Muscle Mass and Strength. J Strength Cond Res; 2018.

194. Refalo MC et al. Influence of Resistance Training Proximity–to–Failure on Skeletal Muscle Hypertrophy: A Systematic Review with Meta–analysis. Sports Med; 2023.

195. Pareja-Blanco F et al. Effects of velocity loss during resistance training on athletic performance, strength gains and muscle adaptations. Scand J Med Sci Sports; 2017.

196. Schoenfeld BJ, Ogborn DI, Vigotsky AD, Franchi MV, Krieger JW. Hypertrophic Effects of Concentric vs. Eccentric Muscle Actions: A Systematic Review and Meta-analysis. J Strength Cond Res; 2017.

197. Tesch PA, Fernandez-Gonzalo R, Lundberg TR. Clinical applications of iso-inertial, eccentric-overload (YoYoTM) resistance exercise. Front Physiol; 2017.

198. Simão R et al. Exercise order in resistance training. Sports Med; 2012.

199. Nuckols G. Periodization: What the Data Say. Stronger by science; 2018.

200. Hayes LD, Bickerstaff GF, Baker JS. Interactions of cortisol, testosterone, and resistance training: Influence of circadian rhythms. Chronobiol Int; 2010.

201. Souissi N, Gauthier A, Sesboüé B, Larue J, Davenne D. Effects of regular training at the same time of day on diurnal fluctuations in muscular performance. J Sports Sci; 2002.

202. Sedliak M, Finni T, Cheng S, Lind M, Häkkinen K. Effect of time-of-day-specific strength training on muscular hypertrophy in men. J Strength Cond Res Natl Strength Cond Assoc; 2009.

203. Sedliak M et al. Morphological, molecular and hormonal adaptations to early morning versus afternoon resistance training. Chronobiol Int; 2018.

204. Schoenfeld BJ et al. Differential effects of attentional focus strategies during long-term resistance training. Eur J Sport Sci; 2018.

205. Tesch P. Muscle Meets Magnet; 1993.

206. Hernández-Belmonte A, Martínez-Cava A, Buendía-Romero Á, Franco-López F, Pallarés JG. Free-Weight and Machine-Based Training Are Equally Effective on Strength and Hypertrophy: Challenging a Traditional Myth. Med Sci Sports Exerc; 2023.

207. Scott BR, Loenneke JP, Slattery KM, Dascombe BJ. Blood flow restricted exercise for athletes: A review of available evidence. J Sci Med Sport; 2016.

208. Pearson SJ, Hussain SR. A Review on the Mechanisms of Blood-Flow Restriction Resistance Training-Induced Muscle Hypertrophy. Sports Med; 2015.

209. Marín PJ, Rhea MR. Effects of vibration training on muscle strength: A meta-analysis. J Strength Cond Res; 2010.

210. Marín PJ, Rhea MR. Effects of vibration training on muscle power: A meta-analysis. J Strength Cond Res; 2010.

211. Morton RW et al. A systematic review, meta-analysis and meta-regression of the effect of protein supplementation on resistance training-induced gains in muscle mass and strength in healthy adults. Br J Sports Med; 2018.

212. Moore DR et al. Differential stimulation of myofibrillar and sarcoplasmic protein synthesis with protein ingestion at rest and after resistance exercise. J Physiol; 2009.

213. Macnaughton LS et al. The response of muscle protein synthesis following whole-body resistance exercise is greater following 40 g than 20 g of ingested whey protein. Physiol Rep; 2016.

214. Moore DR et al. Protein ingestion to stimulate myofibrillar protein synthesis requires greater relative protein intakes in healthy older versus younger men. J Gerontol Ser Biol Sci Med Sci; 2015.

215. Pennings B et al. Whey protein stimulates postprandial muscle protein accretion more effectively than do casein and casein hydrolysate in older men. Am J Clin Nutr; 2011.

216. van Vliet S, Burd NA, van Loon LJ. The Skeletal Muscle Anabolic Response to Plant- versus Animal-Based Protein Consumption. J Nutr; 2015.

217. Phillips SM, Tang JE, Moore DR. The role of milk- and soy-based protein in support of muscle protein synthesis and muscle protein accretion in young and elderly persons. J Am Coll Nutr; 2009.

218. Hevia-Larraín V et al. High-Protein Plant-Based Diet Versus a Protein-Matched Omnivorous Diet to Support Resistance Training Adaptations: A Comparison Between Habitual Vegans and Omnivores. Sports Med; 2021.

219. Koopman R et al. Coingestion of carbohydrate with protein does not further augment postexercise muscle protein synthesis. Am J Physiol Endocrinol Metab; 2007.

220. Gorissen SHM et al. Co-ingesting milk fat with micellar casein does not affect postprandial protein handling in healthy older men. Clin Nutr; 2017.

221. Burd NA et al. Enhanced Amino Acid Sensitivity of Myofibrillar Protein Synthesis Persists for up to 24 h after Resistance Exercise in Young Men. J Nutr; 2011.

222. Burd NA, Beals JW, Martinez IG, Salvador AF, Skinner SK. Food-First Approach to Enhance the Regulation of Post-exercise Skeletal Muscle Protein Synthesis and Remodeling. Sports Med; 2019.

223. Trommelen J, van Loon LJC. Pre-sleep protein ingestion to improve the skeletal muscle adaptive response to exercise training. Nutrients; 2016.

224. Shirvani H et al. The Impact of Pre-sleep Protein Ingestion on the Skeletal Muscle Adaptive Response to Exercise in Humans: An Update. Front Nutr; 2019.

225. Delimaris I. Adverse Effects Associated with Protein Intake above the Recommended Dietary Allowance for Adults. ISRN Nutr; 2013.

226. Van Elswyk ME, Weatherford CA, Mcneill SH. A systematic review of renal health in healthy individuals associated with protein intake above the US recommended daily allowance in randomized controlled trials and observational studies. Adv Nutr; 2018.

227. Antonio J et al. A High Protein Diet Has No Harmful Effects: A One-Year Crossover Study in Resistance-Trained Males. J Nutr Metab; 2016.

228. Maughan RJ et al. IOC consensus statement: Dietary supplements and the high-performance athlete. Int J Sport Nutr Exerc Metab; 2018.

229. Antonio J et al. Common questions and misconceptions about creatine supplementation: what does the scientific evidence really show? J Int Soc Sports Nutr; 2021.

230. Geyer H et al. Analysis of Non-Hormonal Nutritional Supplements for Anabolic-Androgenic Steroids – Results of an International Study. Int J Sports Med; 2004.

231. Deldicque L, Francaux M. Potential harmful effects of dietary supplements in sports medicine. Curr Opin Clin Nutr Metab Care; 2016.

232. Taylor JL, Amann M, Duchateau J, Meeusen R, Rice CL. Neural contributions to muscle fatigue: From the brain to the muscle and back again. Med Sci Sports Exerc; 2016.

233. Chandler JV, Blair SN. The effect of amphetamines on selected physiological components related to athletic success. Med Sci Sports Exerc; 1980.

234. Rollo I, Williams C. Effect of mouth-rinsing carbohydrate solutions on endurance performance. Sports Med; 2011.

235. Allen DG, Lamb GD, Westerblad H. Skeletal Muscle Fatigue: Cellular Mechanisms. Physiol Rev; 2008.

236. Nordsborg N et al. Muscle interstitial potassium kinetics during intense exhaustive exercise: effect of previous arm exercise. Am J Physiol Regul Integr Comp Physiol; 2003.

237. Zhang SJ et al. Limited oxygen diffusion accelerates fatigue development in mouse skeletal muscle. J Physiol; 2006.

238. Dahlstedt AJ, Katz A, Wieringa BÉ, Westerblad H. Is creatine kinase responsible for fatigue? Studies of isolated skeletal muscle deficient in creatine kinase. FASEB J; 2000.

239. Dahlstedt AJ et al. Creatine kinase injection restores contractile function in creatine–kinase–deficient mouse skeletal muscle fibres. J Physiol; 2003.

240. Chin ER, Allen DG. Effects of reduced muscle glycogen concentration on force, Ca2+release and contractile protein function in intact mouse skeletal muscle. J Physiol; 1997.

241. Nielsen J et al. Subcellular distribution of glycogen and decreased tetanic Ca^{2+} in fatigued single intact mouse muscle fibres. J Physiol; 2014.

242. Rai A, Bhati P, Anand P. Exercise induced muscle damage and repeated bout effect: an update for last 10 years and future perspectives. Comp Exerc Physiol; 2023.

243. McHugh MP. Recent advances in the understanding of the repeated bout effect: the protective effect against muscle damage from a single bout of eccentric exercise. Scand J Med Sci Sports; 2003.

244. Owens DJ et al. Exercise–induced muscle damage: What is it, what causes it and what are the nutritional solutions? Eur J Sport Sci; 2018.

245. Morgan DL, Proske U. Popping sarcomere hypothesis explains stretch–induced muscle damage. Clin Exp Pharmacol Physiol; 2004.

246. Ranchordas MK et al. Antioxidants for preventing and reducing muscle soreness after exercise: A Cochrane systematic review. Br J Sports Med; 2018.

247. Versey NG, Halson SL, Dawson B. Water immersion recovery for athletes: Effect on exercise performance and practical recommendations. Sports Med; 2013.

248. Broatch JR, Petersen A, Bishop DJ. The Influence of Post–Exercise Cold–Water Immersion on Adaptive Responses to Exercise: A Review of the Literature. Sports Med; 2018.

249. Cheng AJ et al. Post–exercise recovery of contractile function and endurance in humans and mice is accelerated by heating and slowed by cooling skeletal muscle. J Physiol; 2017.

250. Roberts LA et al. Post–exercise cold water immersion attenuates acute anabolic signalling and long–term adaptations in muscle to strength training. J Physiol; 2015.

251. Fuchs CJ et al. Postexercise cooling impairs muscle protein synthesis rates in recreational athletes. J Physiol; 2020.

252. Paulsen G et al. Vitamin C and E supplementation alters protein signalling after a strength training session, but not muscle growth during 10 weeks of training. J Physiol; 2014.

253. Hernández A, Cheng A, Westerblad H. Antioxidants and Skeletal Muscle Performance: 'Common Knowledge' vs. Experimental Evidence. Front Physiol; 2012.

254. Bjelakovic G, Nikolova D, Gluud C. Antioxidant supplements and mortality. Curr Opin Clin Nutr Metab Care; 2014.

255. Trappe TA et al. Effect of ibuprofen and acetaminophen on postexercise muscle protein synthesis. Am J Physiol Endocrinol Metab; 2002.

256. Mackey AL et al. The influence of anti–inflammatory medication on exercise–induced myogenic precursor cell responses in humans. J Appl Physiol; 2007.

257. Lilja M et al. High doses of anti–inflammatory drugs compromise muscle strength and hypertrophic adaptations to resistance training in young adults. Acta Physiol; 2018.

258. Lilja M et al. Limited effect of over–the–counter doses of ibuprofen on mechanisms regulating muscle hypertrophy during resistance training in young adults. J Appl Physiol; 2023.

259. Brown F et al. Compression Garments and Recovery from Exercise: A Meta–Analysis. Sports Med; 2017.

260. Hickson RC. Interference of strength development by simultaneously training for strength and endurance. Eur J Appl Physiol Occup Physiol; 1980.

261. Schumann M et al. Compatibility of Concurrent Aerobic and Strength Training for Skeletal Muscle Size and Function: An Updated Systematic Review and Meta–Analysis. Sports Med; 2022.

262. Lundberg TR, Feuerbacher JF, Sünkeler M, Schumann M. The Effects of Concurrent Aerobic and Strength Training on Muscle Fiber Hypertrophy: A Systematic Review and Meta–Analysis. Sports Med; 2022.

263. de Souza EO et al. Effects of concurrent strength and endurance training on genes related to myostatin signaling pathway and muscle fiber responses. J Strength Cond Res; 2014.

264. Coffey VG, Hawley JA. Concurrent exercise training: do opposites distract? J Physiol; 2017.

265. Atherton PJ et al. Selective activation of AMPK–PGC–1alpha or PKB–TSC2–mTOR signaling can explain specific adaptive responses to endurance or resistance training–like electrical muscle stimulation. FASEB J; 2005.

266. Lundberg TR et al. Aerobic Exercise Alters Skeletal Muscle Molecular Responses to Resistance Exercise. Med Sci Sports Exerc; 2012.

267. Lundberg TR, Fernandez–Gonzalo R, Tesch PA. Exercise–induced AMPK activation does not interfere with muscle hypertrophy in response to resistance training in men. J Appl Physiol; 2014.

268. Leveritt M, Abernethy PJ, Barry BK, Logan P. Concurrent strength and endurance training. A review. Sports Med; 1999.

269. Petré H et al. Development of Maximal Dynamic Strength During Concurrent Resistance and Endurance Training in Untrained, Moderately Trained, and Trained Individuals: A Systematic Review and Meta–analysis. Sports Med; 2021.

270. Murawska–Cialowicz E, Wojna J, Zuwala–Jagiello J. The physiological effects of concurrent strength and endurance training sequence: A systematic review and meta–analysis. J Sports Sci; 2018.

271. Häkkinen K et al. Neuromuscular adaptations during concurrent strength and endurance training versus strength training. Eur J Appl Physiol; 2003.

272. Bishop D et al. Muscle activation of the knee extensors following high intensity endurance exercise in cyclists. Eur J Appl Physiol; 2000.

273. Leveritt M, Abernethy PJ. Acute Effects of High–Intensity Endurance Exercise on Subsequent Resistance Activity. J Strength Cond Res; 1999.

274. Spiliopoulou P et al. Effect of Concurrent Power Training and High–Intensity Interval Cycling on Muscle Morphology and Performance. J Strength Cond Res; 2021.

275. Aagaard P, Andersen JL. Effects of strength training on endurance capacity in top-level endurance athletes. Scand J Med Sci Sports; 2010.

276. Beattie K et al. The Effect of Strength Training on Performance in Endurance Athletes. Sports Med; 2014.

277. Jones AM. Running economy is negatively related to sit–and–reach test performance in international–standard distance runners. Int J Sports Med; 2002.

278. Paavolainen L et al. Explosive–strength training improves 5–km running time by improving running economy and muscle power. J Appl Physiol; 1999.

279. Hoff J et al. Maximal strength training improves aerobic endurance performance. Scand J Med Sci Sports; 2002.

280. Kraschnewski JL et al. Is strength training associated with mortality benefits? A 15 year cohort study of US older adults. Prev Med; 2016.

281. Abou Sawan S et al. The Health Benefits of Resistance Exercise: Beyond Hypertrophy and Big Weights. Exerc Sport Mov; 2023.

282. Booth FW et al. Role of Inactivity in Chronic Diseases: Evolutionary Insight and Pathophysiological Mechanisms. Physiol Rev; 2017.

283. Pedersen BK, Saltin B. Exercise as medicine – Evidence for prescribing exercise as therapy in 26 different chronic diseases. Scand J Med Sci Sports; 2015.

284. Garcia–Hermoso A et al. Adherence to aerobic and muscle–strengthening activities guidelines: a systematic review and meta–analysis of 3.3 million participants across 32 countries. Br J Sports Med; 2023.

285. Powell KE et al. The Scientific Foundation for the Physical Activity Guidelines for Americans , 2nd Edition. Hum Kinet J; 2019.

286. Artero EG et al. Effects of muscular strength on cardiovascular risk factors and prognosis. J Cardiopulm Rehabil Prev; 2012.

287. Inder JD et al. Isometric exercise training for blood pressure management: A systematic review and meta–analysis to optimize benefit. Hypertens Res; 2016.

288. Snowling NJ, Hopkins WG. Effects of different modes of exercise training on glucose control and risk factors for complications in type 2 diabetic patients: A meta–analysis. Diabetes Care; 2006.

289. Martin SA et al. Highly favorable physiological responses to concurrent resistance and high–intensity interval training during chemotherapy: the OptiTrain breast cancer trial. Breast Cancer Res Treat; 2018.

290. Martin SA et al. Exercise training during chemotherapy preserves skeletal muscle fiber area, capillarization, and mitochondrial content in patients with breast cancer. FASEB J; 2018.

291. Börjesson M. in FYSS (in Swedish): Fysisk aktivitet i sjukdomsprevention och sjukdomsbehandling. Läkartidningen Förlag AB; 2017.

292. Li Z et al. The effect of resistance training on cognitive function in the older adults: a systematic review of randomized clinical trials. Aging Clin Exp Res; 2018.

293. Fernandez–Gonzalo R et al. Muscle, functional and cognitive adaptations after flywheel resistance training in stroke patients: A pilot randomized controlled trial. J NeuroEngineering Rehabil; 2016.

294. Hernlund E et al. Osteoporosis in the European Union: Medical management, epidemiology and economic burden: A report prepared in collaboration with the International Osteoporosis Foundation (IOF) and the European Federation of Pharmaceutical Industry Associations (EFPIA). Arch Osteoporos; 2013.

295. Wright NC et al. The recent prevalence of osteoporosis and low bone mass in the United States based on bone mineral density at the femoral neck or lumbar spine. J Bone Miner; 2014.

296. Suominen H. Muscle training for bone strength. Aging Clin Exp Res; 2006.

297. Karlsson M. Is exercise of value in the prevention of fragility fractures in men? Scand J Med Sci Sports; 2002.

298. Sherrington C et al. Exercise for preventing falls in older people living in the community. Cochrane Database Syst Rev; 2019.

299. King NA et al. Individual variability following 12 weeks of supervised exercise: Identification and characterization of compensation for exercise-induced weight loss. Int J Obes; 2008.

300. Doucet E et al. Evidence for the existence of adaptive thermogenesis during weight loss. Br J Nutr; 2001.

301. Johns DJ, Hartmann-Boyce J, Jebb SA, Aveyard P. Diet or exercise interventions vs combined behavioral weight management programs: A systematic review and meta-analysis of direct comparisons. J Acad Nutr Diet; 2014.

302. Longland TM, Oikawa SY, Mitchell CJ, Devries MC, Phillips SM. High protein exercise caloric restriction promotes greater lean mass gain and fat mass loss. Am J Clin Nutr; 2016.

303. Hector AJ et al. Pronounced energy restriction with elevated protein intake results in no change in proteolysis and reductions in skeletal muscle protein synthesis that are mitigated by resistance exercise. FASEB J; 2018.

304. Volpato S et al. Prevalence and clinical correlates of sarcopenia in community-dwelling older people: Application of the EWGSOP definition and diagnostic algorithm. J Gerontol Ser Biol Sci Med Sci; 2014.

305. Linge J, Dahlqvist Leinhard O. On the definition of sarcopenic obesity – Initial results from UK Biobank. J Gerontol Biol Sci Med Sci; 2019.

306. Deschenes MR. Effects of aging on muscle fibre type and size. Sports Med; 2004.

307. Liguori I et al. Sarcopenia: Assessment of disease burden and strategies to improve outcomes. Clin Interv Aging; 2018.

308. Piasecki M et al. Failure to expand the motor unit size to compensate for declining motor unit numbers distinguishes sarcopenic from non-sarcopenic older men. J Physiol; 2018.

309. Lavretsky H, Newhouse PA. Stress, inflammation, and aging. Am J Geriatr Psychiatry; 2012.

310. Marzetti E et al. Mitochondrial dysfunction and sarcopenia of aging: From signaling pathways to clinical trials. Int J Biochem Cell Biol; 2013.

311. Trappe S et al. New records in aerobic power among octogenarian lifelong endurance athletes. J Appl Physiol; 2013.

312. Hengeveld LM et al. Prevalence of protein intake below recommended in community-dwelling older adults: a meta-analysis across cohorts from the PROMISS consortium. J Cachexia Sarcopenia Muscle; 2020.

313. Nowson C, O'Connell S. Protein Requirements and Recommendations for Older People: A Review. Nutrients; 2015.

314. Robinson K et al. Effects of Resistance Training on Academic Outcomes in School-Aged Youth: A Systematic Review and Meta-Analysis. Sports Med; 2023.

315. Baranto A et al. Back pain and MRI changes in the thoraco-lumbar spine of top athletes in four different sports: A 15-year follow-up study. Knee Surg Sports Traumatol Arthrosc; 2009.

316. Christou M. Effects of resistance training on the physical capacities of adolescent soccer players. J Strength Cond Res; 2006.

317. Lloyd RS et al. Position statement on youth resistance training: The 2014 International Consensus. Br J Sports Med; 2014.

318. Faigenbaum AD, Myer GD. Resistance training among young athletes: Safety, efficacy and injury prevention effects. Br J Sports Med; 2010.

319. Myer GD, et al. Youth versus adult "weightlifting" injuries presenting to United States emergency rooms: accidental versus nonaccidental injury mechanisms. J Strength Cond Res; 2009.

320. Falk B, Tenenbaum G. The effectiveness of resistance training in children. A meta-analysis. Sports Med; 1996.

321. Fukunaga T et al. The effects of resistance training on muscle area and strength in prepubescent age. Ann Physiol Anthr; 1992.

322. Moran J et al. A Meta-Analysis of Resistance Training in Female Youth: Its Effect on Muscular Strength, and Shortcomings in the Literature. Sports Med; 2018.

323. Behringer M et al. Effects of resistance training in children and adolescents: a meta-analysis. Pediatrics; 2010.

324. Johnson DM et al. The influence of exposure, growth and maturation on injury risk in male academy football players. J Sports Sci; 2022.

325. Hilton EN, Lundberg TR. Transgender Women in the Female Category of Sport: Perspectives on Testosterone Suppression and Performance Advantage. Sports Med; 2021.

326. Nuzzo JL. Narrative Review of Sex Differences in Muscle Strength, Endurance, Activation, Size, Fiber Type, and Strength Training Participation Rates, Preferences, Motivations, Injuries, and Neuromuscular Adaptations. J Strength Cond Res; 2023.

327. Kataoka R et al. Sex segregation in strength sports: Do equal-sized muscles express the same levels of strength between sexes? Am J Hum Biol; 2023.

328. Essen-Gustavsson B, Borges O. Histochemical and metabolic characteristics of human skeletal muscle in relation to age. Acta Physiol Scand; 1986.

329. Jansson E, Hedberg G. Skeletal muscle fibre types in teenagers: relationship to physical performance and activity. Scand J Med Sci Sports; 1991.

330. Nottelmann ED et al. Developmental processes in early adolescence. Relations among chronologic age, pubertal stage, height, weight, and serum levels of gonadotropins, sex steroids, and adrenal androgens. J Adolesc Health Care; 1987.

331. Kraemer WJ, Ratamess NA. Hormonal responses and adaptations to resistance exercise and training. Sports Med; 2005.

332. Wang X et al. Testosterone increases the muscle protein synthesis rate but does not affect very-low-density lipoprotein metabolism in obese premenopausal women. Am J Physiol Endocrinol Metab; 2012.

333. West DW et al. Sex-based comparisons of myofibrillar protein synthesis after resistance exercise in the fed state. J Appl Physiol; 2012.

334. Smith GI, Mittendorfer B. Similar muscle protein synthesis rates in young men and women: men aren't from Mars and women aren't from Venus. J Appl Physiol; 2012.

335. Colenso-Semple LM et al. Current evidence shows no influence of women's menstrual cycle phase on acute strength performance or adaptations to resistance exercise training. Front Sports Act Living; 2023.

336. Samson M. Relationships between physical performance measures, age, height and body weight in healthy adults. Age Ageing; 2000.

337. Sørensen MB et al. Obesity and sarcopenia after menopause are reversed by sex hormone replacement therapy. Obes Res; 2001.

338. Greising SM et al. Hormone therapy and skeletal muscle strength: A meta-analysis. J Gerontol Ser Biol Sci Med Sci; 2009.

339.   Hansen M et al. Effects of estrogen replacement and lower androgen status on skeletal muscle collagen and myofibrillar protein synthesis in postmenopausal women. J Gerontol Ser Biol Sci Med Sci; 2012.

340.   Evenson KR, Wen F. National trends in self–reported physical activity and sedentary behaviors among pregnant women: NHANES 1999–2006. Prev Med; 2010.

341.   Downs DS et al. Physical Activity and Pregnancy: Past and Present Evidence and Future Recommendations. Res Quaterly Exerc Sport; 2012.

342.   Ravanelli N et al. Heat stress and fetal risk. Environmental limits for exercise and passive heat stress during pregnancy: a systematic review with best evidence synthesis. Br J Sports Med; 2019.

343.   FYSS (in Swedish): Fysisk aktivitet i sjukdomsprevention och sjukdomsbehandling. Läkartidningen Förlag AB; 2017.

344.   O'Connor PJ et al. Safety and Efficacy of Supervised Strength Training Adopted in Pregnancy. J Phys Act Health; 2011.

345.   Perales M et al. Benefits of aerobic or resistance training during pregnancy on maternal health and perinatal outcomes: A systematic review. Early Hum Dev; 2016.

346.   Young WB. Transfer of strength and power training to sports performance. Int J Sports Physiol Perform; 2006.

Printed in Great Britain
by Amazon